# Tai Chi for Health

## The 24 Simplified Forms

Cheng Zhao
Don Zhao

*Agilceed Books*
*Indiana, U.S.A.*

TITILE Tai Chi for Health: The 24 Simplified Forms

ISBN 0-976118-31-9

Special quantity discount or sample copies for promotional sales may be available from Agilceed Books. For more information, please write to the Sales Manager, Educational Publishing, Agilceed Books at 309 Woodbine Drive, Terre Haute, IN 47803. For information on bulk purchase prices, translations or book distributors outside the U.S.A., please contact Agilceed Books at agilceed@gmail.com.

March, 2006

# Acknowledgment

We would like to express our gratefulness to Mr. Robert Watson, a long time Tai Chi practitioner, who spent his valuable time reviewing the manuscript of this book carefully. His valuable suggestions and corrections make this book better source of reference. We would also like to thank grandmaster Li Guang Qi for allowing us to publish his images of Tai Chi postures. This book would not be complete without his help.

# Tai Chi for Health

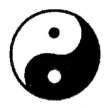

## Table of Contents

## What is Tai Chi Chuan?

*Tai Chi Chuan is one of the classic Chinese martial arts that was passed down generations after generations. It has now developed into a supreme method for improving mental health, physical fitness, and spiritual growth for people at any age.*

# Tai Chi for Health

## Inside the physical moves

Tai Chi emphasizes the integrity of body and mind. Ancient in its origin and deep in spiritual roots, Tai Chi Chuan is a type of "moving meditation" that unifies body and

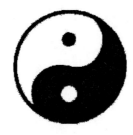

mind. Its movements are graceful and slow, soft and coordinated, continuous and flowing, relaxed and dynamic. It harmonizes body, mind, and spirit.

# Tai Chi for Health

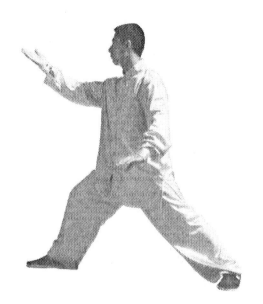

This book is based on authentic Tai Chi Chuan methods that are taught in China today. In using these lessons, a student will learn how to correctly perform each posture, how to use the mind in the performance, and how to correctly regulate the breath. A student will learn the flow of the postures and how to correctly change directions. Special attention will be paid to the transition between each posture.

Tai Chi Chuan is a supreme martial art that has become a supreme method of physical, mental, and spiritual exercise. The study of Tai Chi Chuan is the study of life itself. It is a martial art that can be a life art.

May you enjoy the learning experience of Tai Chi.

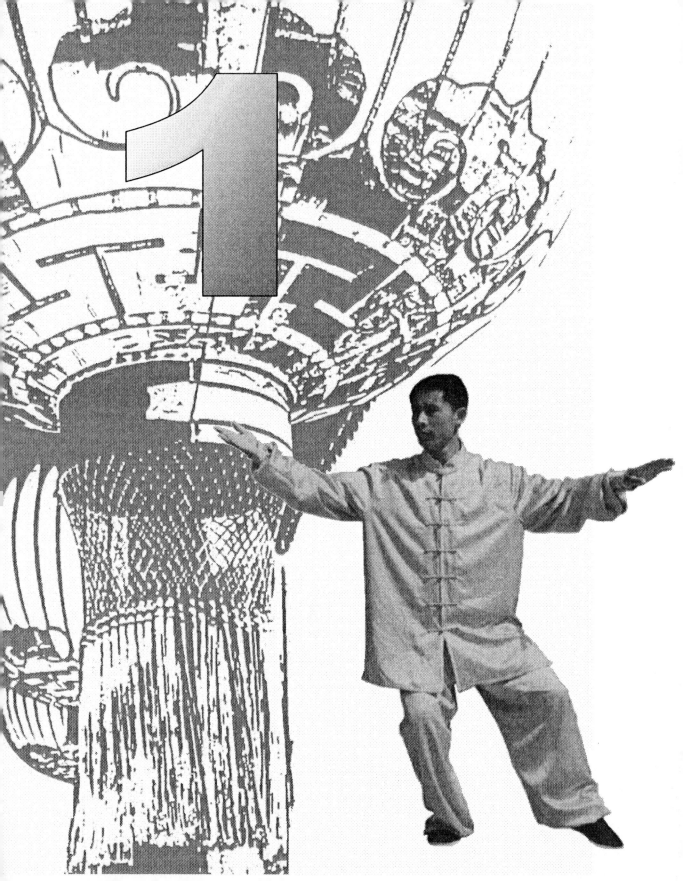

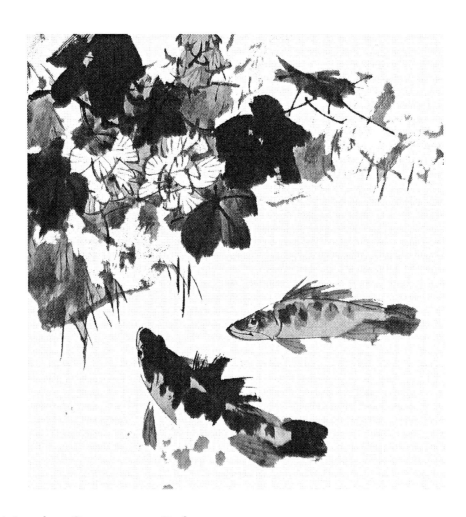

## Tai Chi is the Supreme Pole

Tai Chi Chuan in Chinese is Tai Chi Chuan or Tai Ji Quan, in which Tai Chi is the philosophical notion of the Supreme Pole and Chuan the force. The notion of the Supreme Pole is related to the Chinese concept of yin-yang that interprets natural phenomenon with dynamic duality, the interaction of male and female, darkness and light, force and yield. Chuan is the driving force that moves opposite parts of yin-yang.

# Tai Chi for Health

The word Tai Chi originated from a Chinese ancient book whose title is Yi Jing meaning the principles of nature and its transitions. Tai Chi Chuan carries the philosophies in Yi Jing inside its moves and transitions and thereby has developed into a form of exercise with its own unique style.

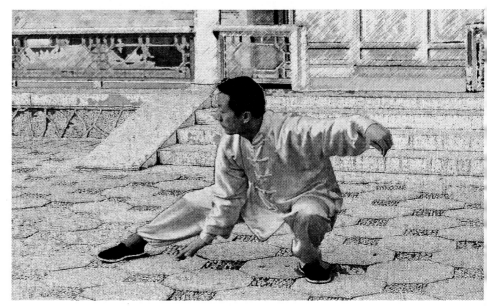

## Is it like Yoga

For many, Tai Chi Chuan practiced in the west is like a moving form of yoga. However, there is more to it inside than the physical movement. The physical exercise of Tai Chi is deeply rooted in philosophical context of Taoism, established by an ancient Chinese scholar named Lao Tsu. Taoism has many elements for the guidance of how to live a better life. Its primary principle resides on a calm and reflective view of the world.

Symbolism was a source of power in Taoist thinking. Symbols form magic diagrams that were regarded as potent talisman having great command over spiritual forces. The core of Tao's symbolism is yin-yang which interplays the eternal exchange of force in a harmonic way to form the divine order of heaven, the integration of the earth and the mankind, and the inner workings of the universe. It is no surprise to find that the symbolism of names has infiltrated the forms of Tai Chi in many ways.

In numerology, Taoists prefer the number '5' and consider it to be a special number with mystical significance. Examples are five emotions, five directions, five elements, five colors, five planets, five mountains, five virtues, and so forth. In Tai Chi we see five Repulse Monkeys or five Wave Hands Like Clouds .

## 5 Xing and 8 Gua

Tai Chi practiced in the East has a long connection with the 5-Xing and 8-Gua, the former of which is five elements of Chinese alchemy (metal, wood, water, fire and earth) and the latter are eight combinations of Yin and Yang.

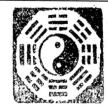

*Tai Chi & 8 Gua*

# Tai Chi for Health

Tai Chi practice as many reach its higher levels of proficiency has drawn the inner power from the deep understanding of all elements of Taoist philosophy, by which the movements become yielding, slow, soft, centered, balanced, and rooted to the ground. These understandings become the principles of Tai Chi and find their ways in both health and martial art applications. One can see the application of these principles in Tai Chi forms like Wave Hands Like Clouds, White Crane Shows Wings, and Repulse the Monkey. Tai Chi works on your body and your mind at the same time. The movements not only relax your muscles, they calm your nerves as well. It is important to understand that the very first lesson of Tai Chi is to relax, which is to yield to the stress and stiffness of your body.

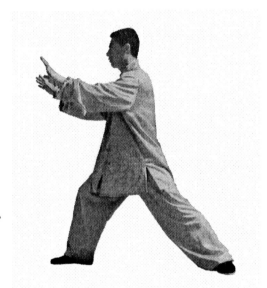

## Lao Tsu, the founder of Taoism, wrote in Tao Te Bible:

| | | |
|---|---|---|
| Yield and overcome; bend and be straight. | Standing on tiptoe is not steady; marching in stride cannot maintain the pace. | What is firmly established cannot be uprooted; what is firmly grasped cannot slip away. |

As a healing art, Tai Chi can be effective in:

1. Improving flexibility, coordination, and concentration;
2. Increasing physical strength and stamina;
3. Relieving stress and pain;
4. Improving concentration and memory;
5. Enhancing sensory awareness;

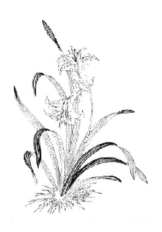

6. Regulating bodily organs naturally;
7. And helping to control a wide range of common chronic ailments such as arthritis, high blood pressure, and heart and respiratory problems.

## Tai Chi is an effective therapy

Nowadays the fast-paced office life often results in stress and lack of sufficient physical activity, which leads to a wide range of health problems, including poor circulation, headaches, high blood pressure, back pain, digestive and nervous disorders, and etc. Many have found the gentle moves, stretching and turning of Tai Chi to be an effective therapy for their health problems.

# Tai Chi for Health

14

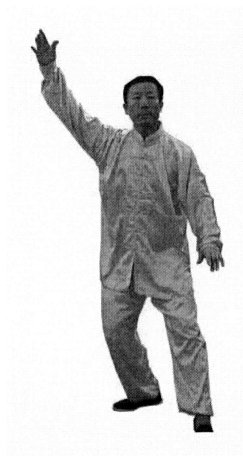

As a physical exercise, Tai Chi Chuan does not emphasize power and muscular force. Rather, Tai Chi Chuan teaches a person to use internal relaxation and awareness to achieve a goal. Following the ancient Chinese philosophy of Yin and Yang, Tai Chi Chuan moves elegantly and gracefully between the seeming opposites of fullness and emptiness, hardness and softness, force and gentleness. Like nature itself, Tai Chi Chuan is constantly seeking balance – flowing like water, never directly opposing any obstacle.

## Stillness is not empty

The interplay of stillness and movement is fundamental to Tai Chi, as it is to life. You will find that each Tai Chi form begins and ends with standing still for a few seconds. Note that this is not an empty pause but an integral part of the Tai Chi practice. The stillness is essential. It is not empty. The stillness allows one to store energy and the movement is connected by stillness.

The foundation of Tai Chi Chuan is the performance of the forms, a series of slow, circular movements based on martial arts postures. They are a pre-choreographed routine of natural movements, practiced slowly and deliberately, using the mind to guide the body.

Each posture is poetic in name as well as execution, for example, Wave Hands Like Clouds, Grasp Peacock's Tail, Hand-hold the Lute, White Crane Shows Wings, and Works at Shuttles.

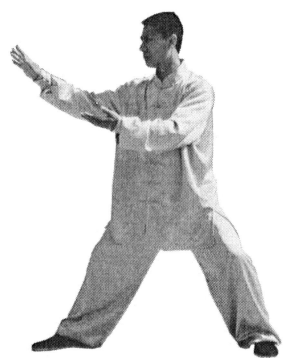

15

## Tai Chi emphasizes the internal energy flow

Tai Chi emphasizes the internal energy flow that penetrates deeper than just the muscles. The messages from Taoism empower the exercise.

Tai Chi benefits the entire physiology of the body by restoring proper circulation and relieving tension in the muscles, ligaments and tendons.

Tai Chi helps optimize the functioning of the body, organs and tissues.

## Tai Chi for Health

There are several major styles of Tai Chi Chuan. These styles named for the families that originated these styles – Chen, Sun, Yang, and Wu. Yang style Tai Chi Chuan is now the most popular style, both in

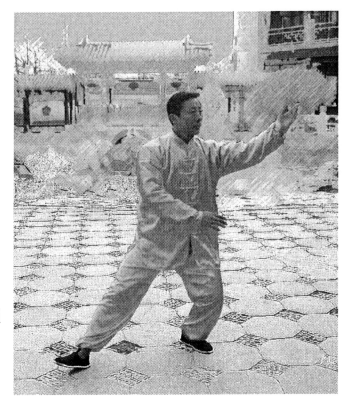

China and the world. It is well known for enhancing the health of its students as well as being an effective martial art. It is suitable for all ages and physical conditions. Because of these advantages, this tutorial will focus on the Yang style of Tai Chi Chuan.

## History of the 24 Simplified Forms

In 1956, the Chinese Sports Committee developed a simplified version of Tai Chi Chuan based primarily on the Yang style. This simplified form is a series of 24 forms that can be performed in about five or six minutes. It was designed as an easily learned series of movements that could be used by anyone to improve their health. Today, the 24 Forms are played by Tai Chi Chuan enthusiasts throughout the world.

16

The basic principles of Yang style are:

1.   Relaxation;

2.   Separation of Yin and Yang (substantial and insubstantial);

3.   All moments are directed and commanded by the waist;

4.   The spine is kept straight and upright;

5.   A focused awareness of slowness, gracefulness, softness, relaxation, and keeping a flowing continuity when executing the forms.

This book presents the 24 Simplified Forms in a tutorial style.  For the student who wants to begin studying Tai Chi Chuan, this is your reference source that will help you learn the Tai Chi forms correctly.

## Making Tai Chi a way of life

To gain the full benefit of Tai Chi, you should consider Tai Chi a way of life, which does not mean you have to practice Tai Chi 24 hours a day, but to develop a habit of thinking and doing it regularly . Tai Chi should become a habit of life by which your physical body is properly aligned while sitting, walking, reading, driving, eating, and even watching TV. Thus you weave Tai Chi into your daily life.

# Tai Chi for Health

However, many cannot learn Tai Chi only from books. Without a qualified teacher, many students are left with incomplete or confusing instructions as to how Tai Chi Chuan is performed. It is not the intention of this book to teach every thing of the 24 Forms, but to be used as a reference to enhance what you get from your current teacher and for the experienced Tai Chi Chuan enthusiasts to study the postures and the connections between moves.

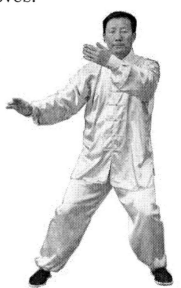

Tai Chi is learned by doing. It takes one or two months to learn the 24 forms. Beginners first learn the forms by mimicking the teacher's demonstration. This allows the students to start with the correct postures and moves. The teacher usually demonstrates a move several times and asks the class to follow. A good teacher will watch for the moves of each student as the class follows along.

## Workload and capacity

When practicing Tai Chi, how much work to do is usually measured by how much time you practice. Use your own judgment for your physical capacity. Unlike other workouts, the amount of your exercise is said to be right if you are comfortable and in high spirit after the practice.

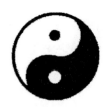

If you are not in great physical shape, don't worry. Tai Chi is for people of all ages and conditions. That is where Tai Chi is different from other workouts. One can practice Tai Chi in comfortable clothing. A good pair of sneakers will help better support and balance. The book divides the 24 forms into 6 groups to help you learn Tai Chi in small steps. Each group of forms can be repeated by itself and then be connected to the next one. The foremost thing for the first time students is to learn Tai Chi moves correctly. Wrong moves and postures will become a habit and difficult to correct. Learn fewer moves if it is difficult to absorb everything taught in a class.

**19**

## Root on foot

The essence of Tai Chi from standing post to combat applications is the root on your foot; that is your connection to the ground. Think of gravity and increase the awareness of how gravity acts upon you. Keep good balance, the earth will pull you down by nature.

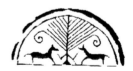

*The nature is simple*
*—Lao Tsu*

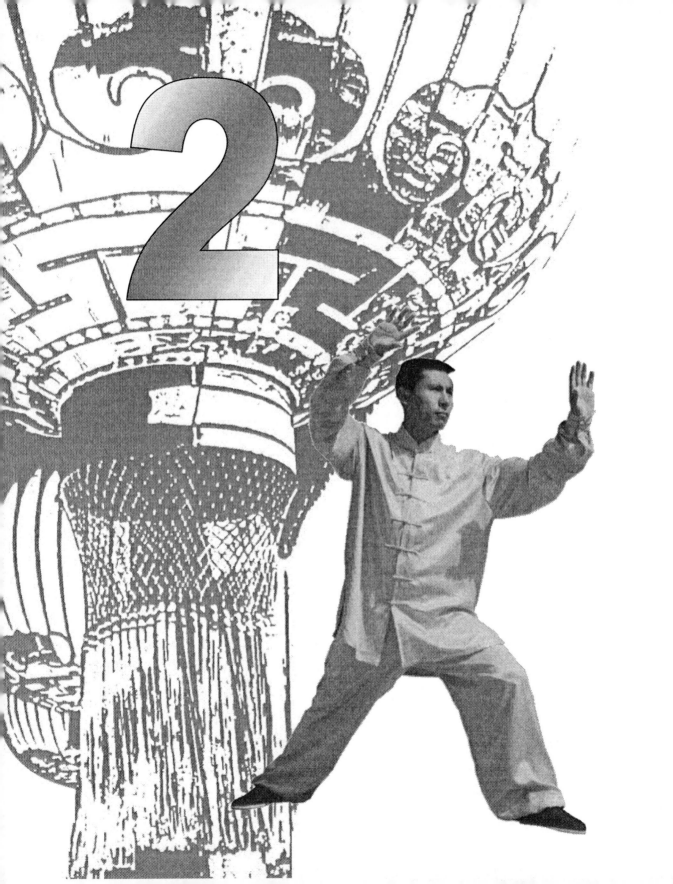

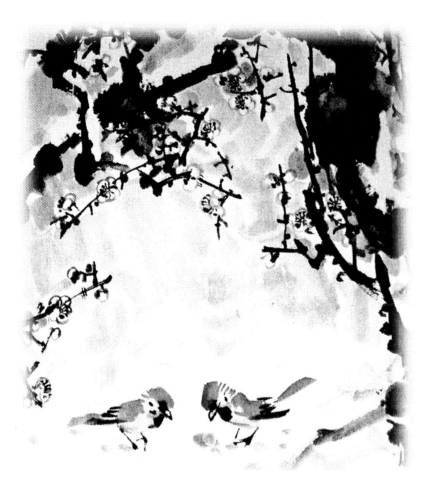

## Beginning from the 24 Forms

The 24 forms were devised as an introduction to the art of
Tai Chi Chuan.  It is the first course for Tai Chi and is used
by many as a starting point to pursue more difficult and
strenuous routines, such as the 32 Sword Forms.  Both routines are taken from Yang Style Tai Chi Chuan.  The 32
Sword Form was choreographed after the 24 Simplified
Forms.

# Tai Chi for Health

| | |
|---|---|
| 01. | Starting Form |
| 02. | Wild Horse Splits Mane (LRL) |
| 03. | White Crane Shows Wings |
| 04. | Brush Knee Turn Steps (LR) |
| 05. | Hand-hold the Lute |
| 06. | Repulse the Monkey (LRLR) |
| 07. | Left Grasp the Peacock's Tail |
| 08. | Right Grasp the Peacock's Tail |
| 09. | Single Whip |
| 10. | Wave Hands Like Clouds |
| 11. | Single Whip |
| 12. | High Hand Pats the Horse |
| 13. | Kick with Right Heel |
| 14. | Strike Ears with Both Fists |
| 15. | Turn and Kick with Left Heel |
| 16. | Left Down One-leg Stand |
| 17. | Right Down One-leg Stand |
| 18. | Works at Shuttles (LR) |
| 19. | Find a Needle at Sea Bottom |
| 20. | Flash Arms |
| 21. | Turn to Deflect, Block, and Strike |
| 22. | Seal as Close-up |
| 23. | Cross Hands |
| 24. | Conclusion |

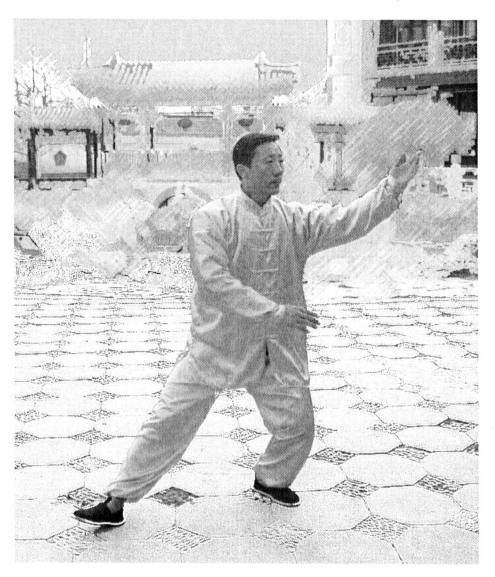

The left side table lists the 24 forms of Tai Chi Moves in the Simplified 24 Forms.  For the ease of learning, we have divided the 24 Forms into six groups with a brief description of each form.  This section can serve as a quick reference once you have learned the 24 Forms.

## Group 1

### Form 1: Starting Form

Form 1 is the beginning form from the standing posture, which we call Starting Form.

[1a]: left foot opens to shoulder width;

[1b]: lift arms and hands to shoulder level and push them to the waist level.

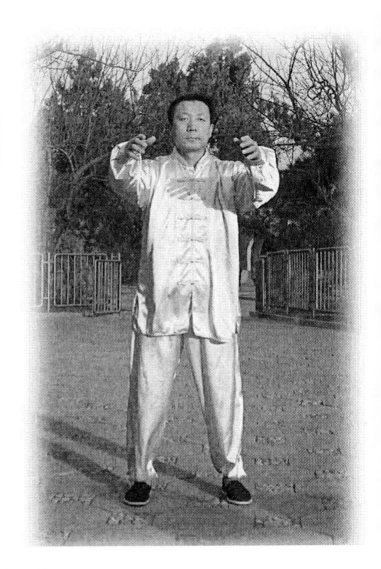

**24**

## Sequence of Form 1 —Starting Form

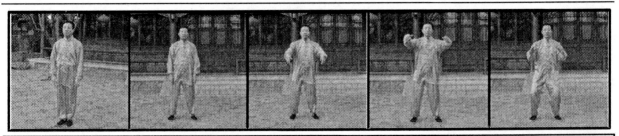

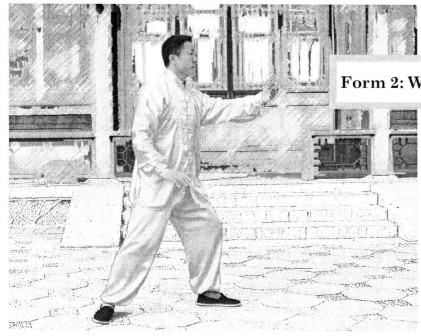

## Group 1

### Form 2: Wild Horse Splits Mane

In Form 2, arms move from center to side three times, first left, then right, and left.

[2a]: left leg, arm & hand move upward and forward, right arm moves backward and downward;

[2b]: right leg, arm & hand move upward and forward, left arm moves backward and downward;
[2c]: left leg, arm & hand move upward and forward, right arm backward and downward.

## Sequence of Form 2 —Wild Horse Splits Mane

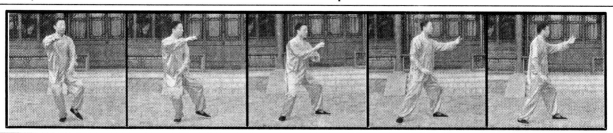

# Tai Chi for Health

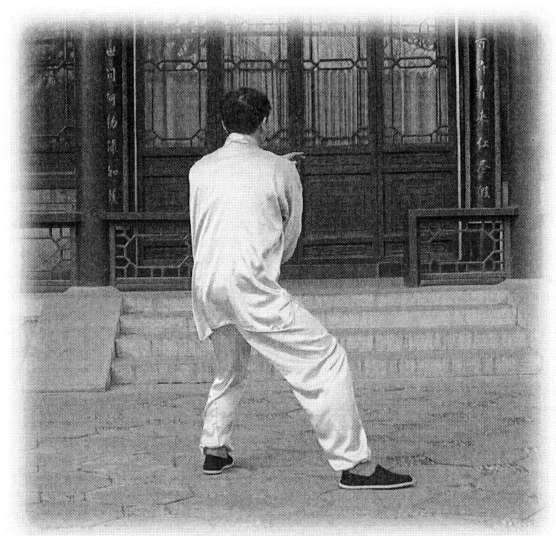

## Sequence of Form 2 Continued

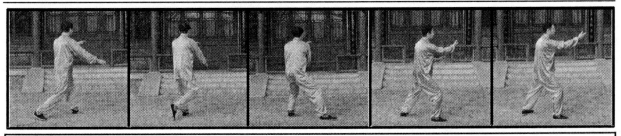

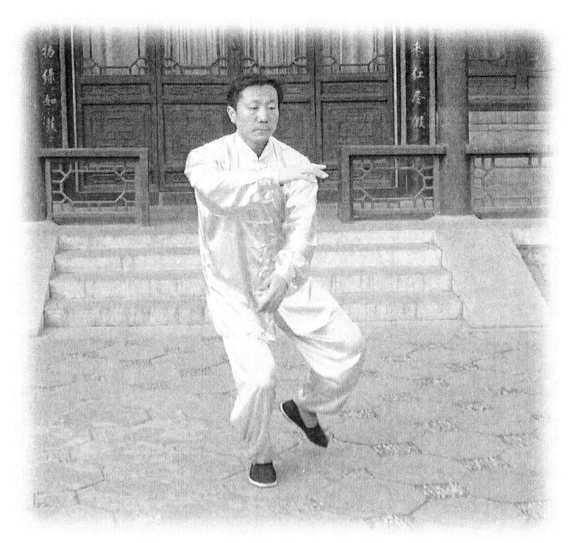

## Sequence of Form 2 Continued

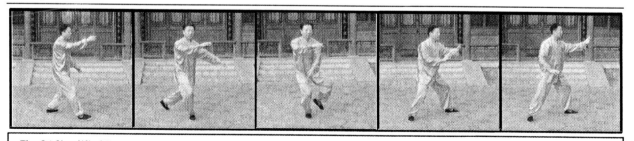

## Form 3: White Crane Shows Wings

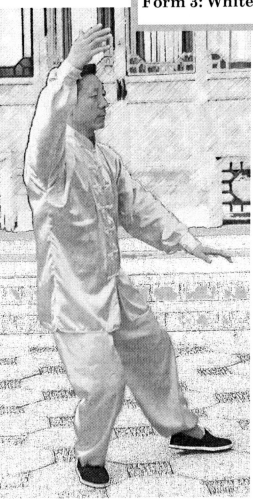

In Form 3, we mimic the shape of a crane with its wings spread out.

[3a]: half step forward, sit on the right leg, and hold a ball in front;

[3b]: separate arms with right hand high, left hand low.

## Sequence of Form 3 —White Crane Shows Wings

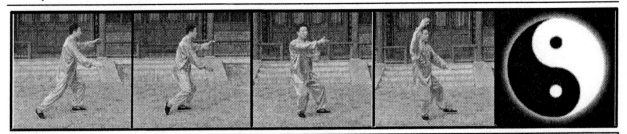

## Group 1

### Form 4: Brush Knee Turn Steps

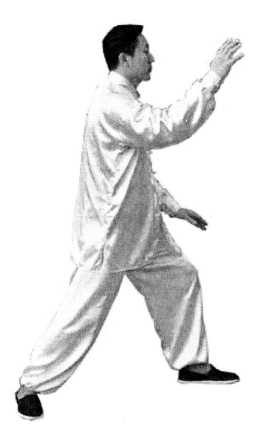

In Form 4, the lower hand moves away from center as if brushing knee. We twist and step forward to help turn the body and push upper hand forward. Repeat the move three times for left, then right, and left sides.

[4a]: left bow stance, left hand brushes left knee, right palm pushes forward;

[4b]: right bow stance, right hand brushes right knee, left palm pushes forward;

[4c]: left bow stance, left hand brushes left knee, right palm pushes forward.

**29**

## Sequence of Form 4 —Brush Knee Turn Steps

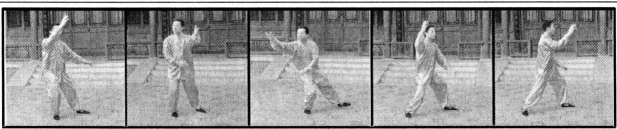

# Tai Chi for Health

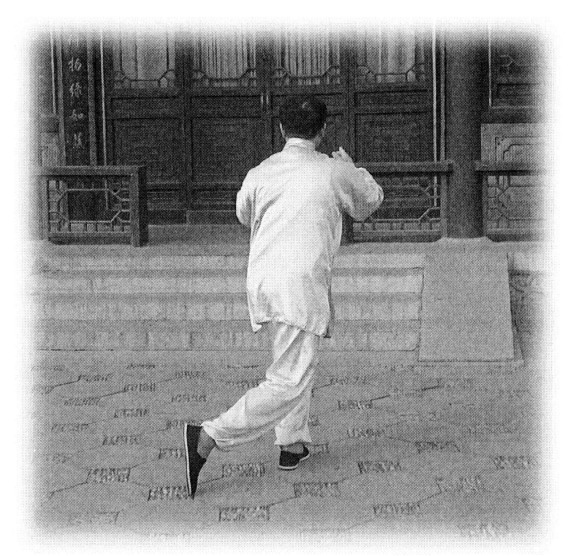

## Sequence of Form 4 Continued

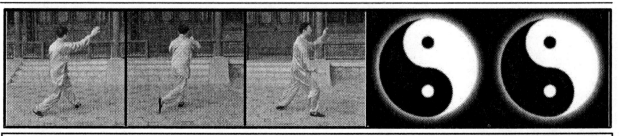

30

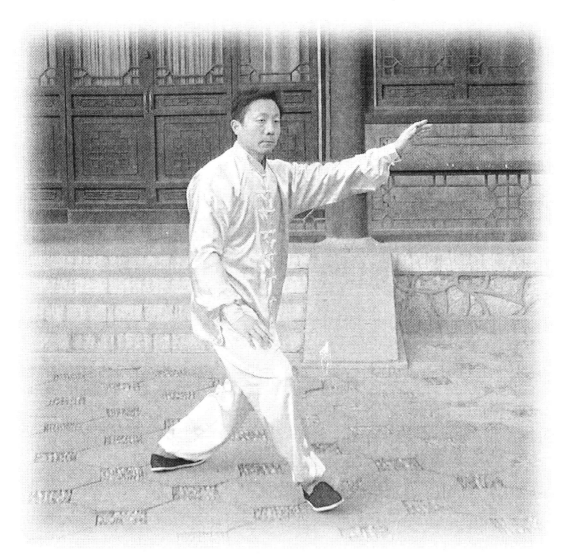

## Sequence of Form 4 Continued

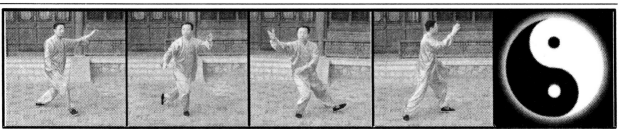

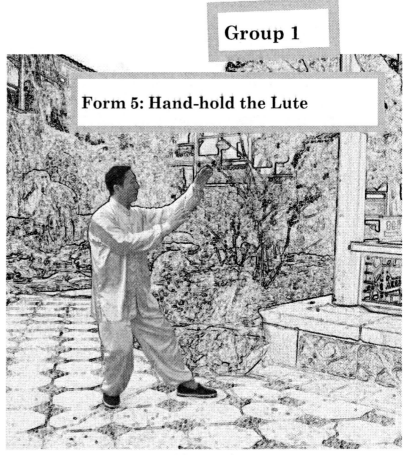

**Group 1**

**Form 5: Hand-hold the Lute**

32

In some books, Form 5 is called "Play the Lute". However, the representative move of this form is like one holding a lute with both arms so that we call it Hand-hold the Lute.

[5a]: half step forward, sit on the right leg;

[5b]: left hand high, right hand low.

## Sequence of Form 5 —Hand-hold the Lute

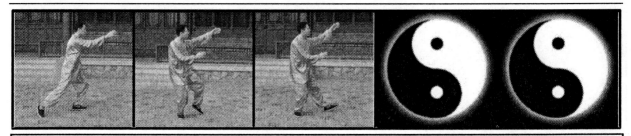

In this form, we step back and push-pull hands in opposite directions. Some trainers would call this form Step Back and Whirl Arm.

**Group 2**

**Form 6: Repulse the Monkey**

33

We call it Repulse Monkey because it is like a monkey retreating. The entire form consists of four sub-routines for left, right, left, and right sides.

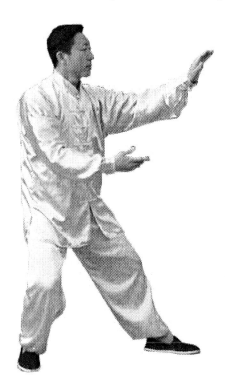

[6a]: pull left leg, arm & hand backward, push right arm & hand forward;

[6b]: pull right leg, arm & hand backward, push left arm & hand forward;

[6c]: pull left leg, arm & hand backward, push right arm & hand forward;

[6d]: pull right leg, arm & hand backward, push left arm & hand forward.

## Sequence of Form 6 —Repulse the Monkey

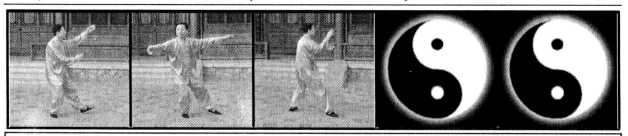

# Tai Chi for Health

## Sequence of Form 6 Continued

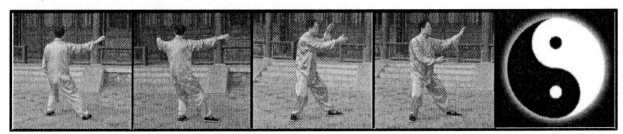

**34**

## Sequence of Form 6 Continued

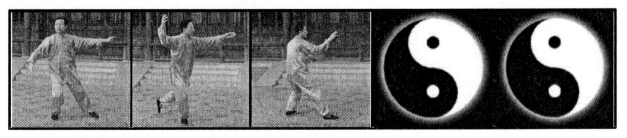

## Sequence of Form 6 Continued

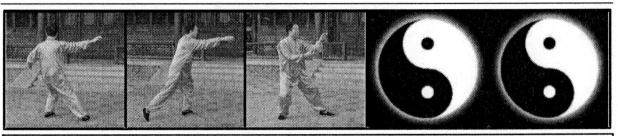

# Chapter 2  The 24 Forms

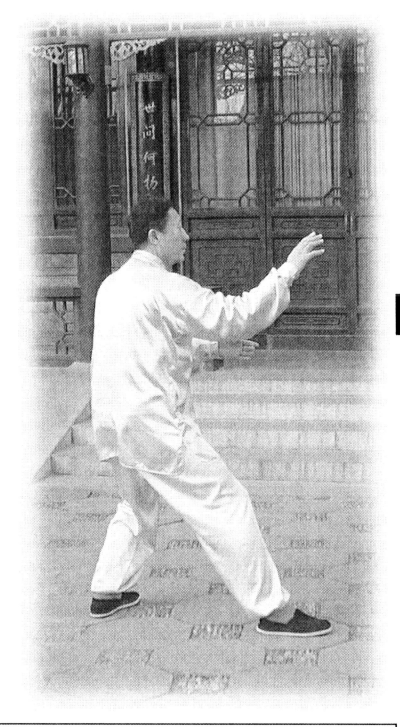

"Grasp the Peacock's Tail" is the largest in the 24 forms. Form 7 is for the left side. It consists of the following four parts:

## Form 7: Left Grasp the Peacock's Tail

[7a]: Ward Off;

[7b]: Roll Back;

[7c]: Press;

[7d]: Push.

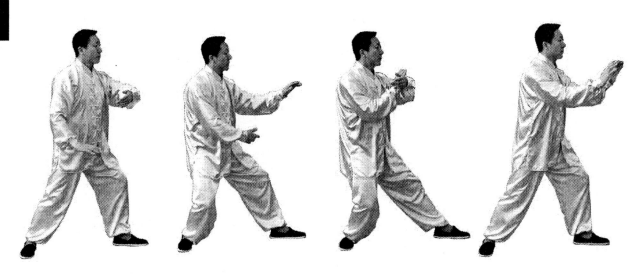

## Sequence of Form 7 —Left grasp the peacock's tail

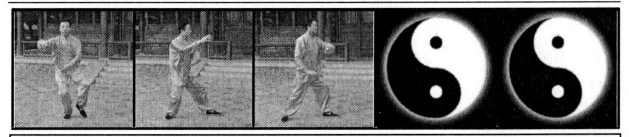

## Sequence of Form 7 Continued

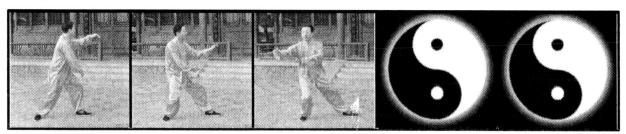

## Sequence of Form 7 Continued

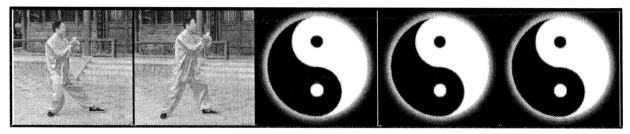

## Sequence of Form 7 Continued

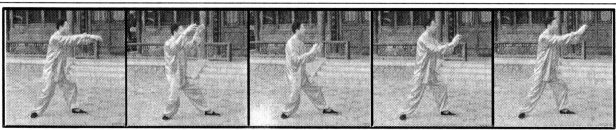

## Sequence of Form 8 —Right Grasp the Peacock's Tail

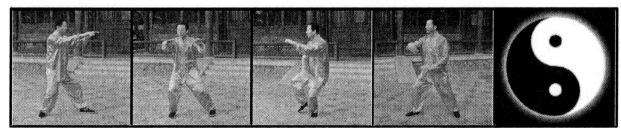

## Sequence of Form 8 Continued

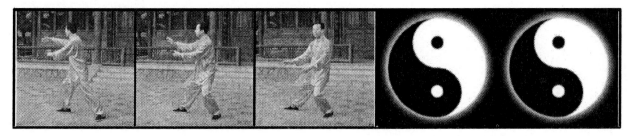

## Sequence of Form 8 Continued

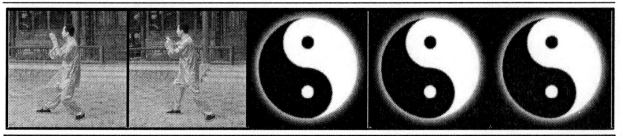

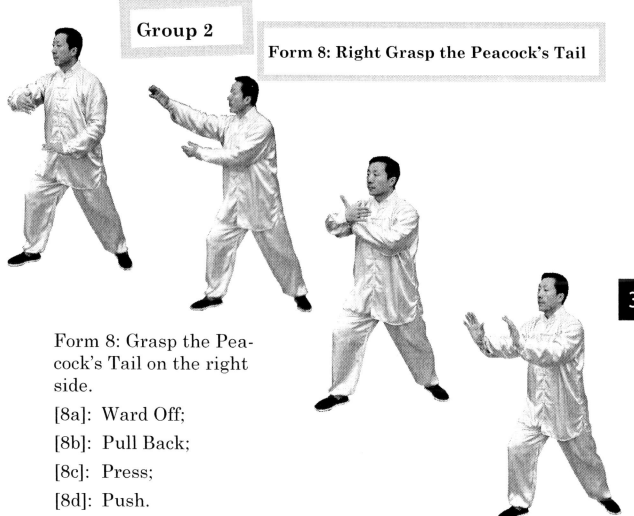

## Group 2

### Form 8: Right Grasp the Peacock's Tail

Form 8: Grasp the Peacock's Tail on the right side.

[8a]:  Ward Off;

[8b]:  Pull Back;

[8c]:  Press;

[8d]:  Push.

## Sequence of Form 8 Continued

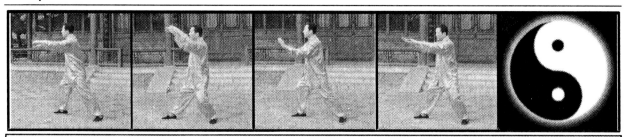

# Tai Chi for Health

Single Whip is completed with a pause of posture as shown below.

[9a]: left foot steps forward into bow stance;

[9b]: right hand in form hook and left hand pushes forward.

**Form 9: Single Whip**

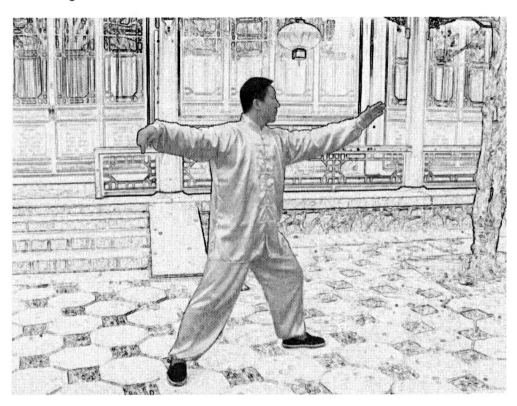

## Sequence of Form 9 —Single Whip

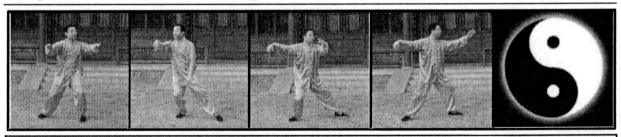

As the name implies, we wave our hands as if we were touching clouds. It is soft, smooth and circular.

[10a]: move from right side to left side, circle arms up and down;

[10b]: move from left side to right side, circle arms up and down;

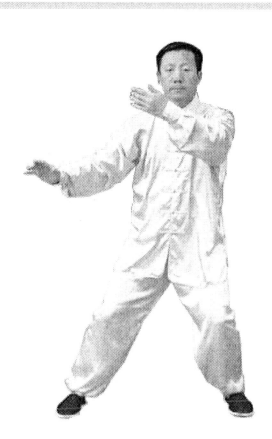

**Group 3**

**Form 10: Wave Hands Like Clouds**

[10c]: move from right side to left side, circle arms up and down;

[10d]: move from left side to right side, circle arms up and down;

[10e]: move from right side to left side, circle arms up and down.

[10f]: move from left side to right side and into the 2nd Single Whip.

41

## Sequence of Form 10 —Wave Hands Like Clouds

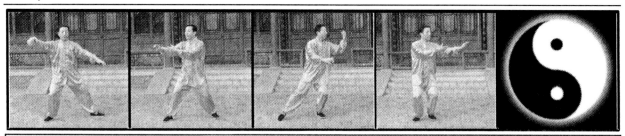

# Tai Chi for Health

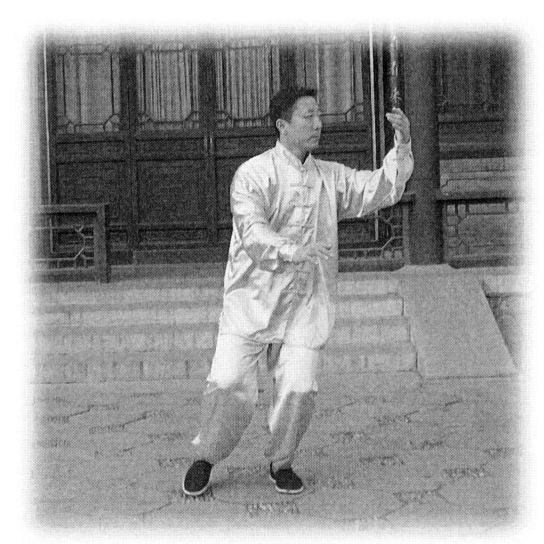

## Sequence of Form 10 Continued

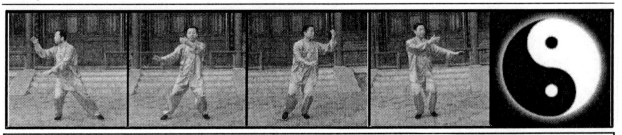

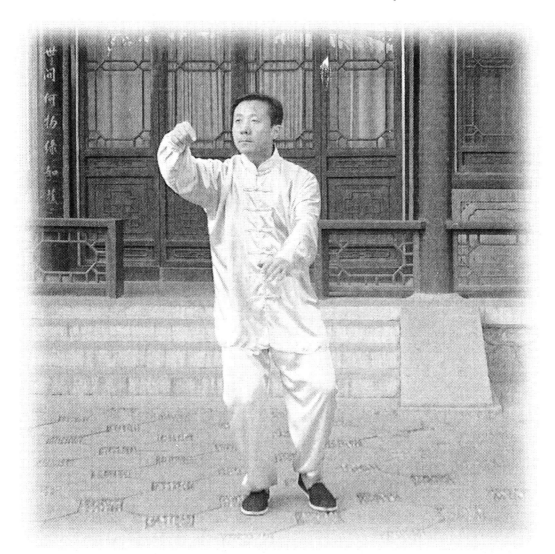

# Sequence of Form 10 Continued

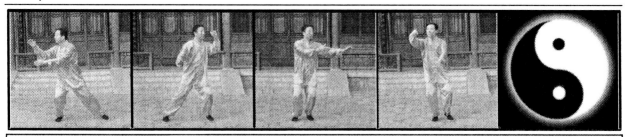

## Group 3

### Form 11: Single Whip

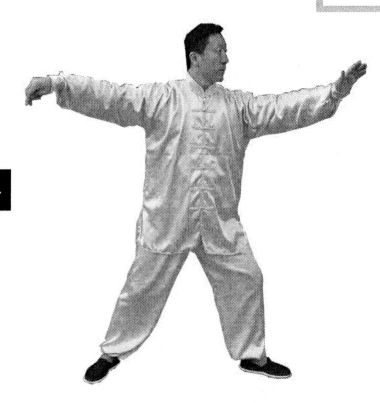

Single Whip in Form 11 is a repeat of Form 9, which is again performed as follows:

[9a]: left foot steps forward into bow stance;

[9b]: right hand in form hook and left hand pushes forward.

## Sequence of Form 11 —Single Whip

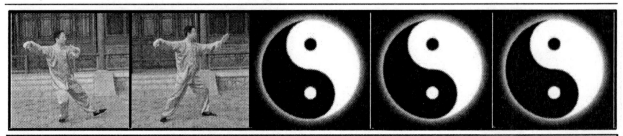

## Group 3

## Form 12: High Hand Pats the Horse

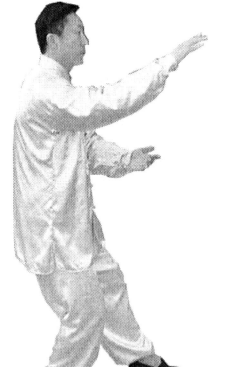

In this form, extend your upper hand (high hand) to pose like patting a horse.  Here is how it is performed.

[12a]: half a step forward, sit on the right leg;

[12b]: right palm pushes forward and up; left hand pulls back and down.

# Sequence of Form 12 —High Hand Pats the Horse

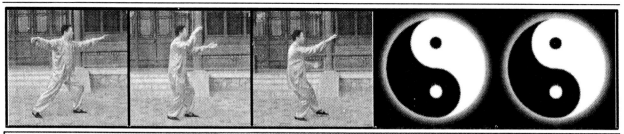

## Group 4

### Form 13: Kick with Right Heel

Form 13 has a slight pause on a right-side while the right foot kicks out with both arms extended out for balance.

46

[13a]: stand on the left leg and lift the right foot;

[13b]: Kick with Right Heel, right arm opens forward at shoulder height while left arm moves back.

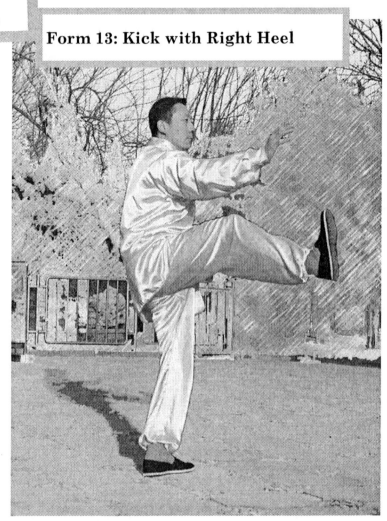

## Sequence of Form 13 —Kick with Right Heel

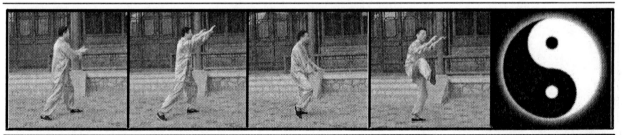

## Group 4

### Form 14: Strike Ears with Both Fists

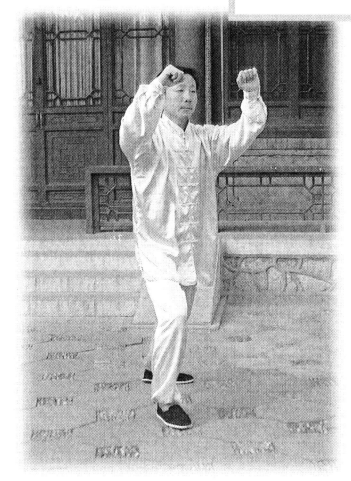

In Form 14, we strike out at the ear level with both fists.

[14a]: step forward in a right bow stance;

[14b]: strike the opponent's ears with both fists.

## Sequence of Form 14 —Strike Ears with Both Fists

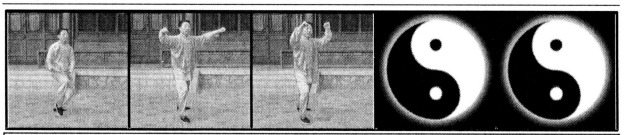

## Group 4

### Form 15: Turn and Kick with Left Heel

Form 15 is a turn followed by a kick with the left heel. We balance on the right foot in this posture for a second or two.

**48**

[15a]: turn your body, cross hands and then separate them in front of the face;

[15b]: kick with left heel; left arm opens forward at shoulder height while right arm moves back.

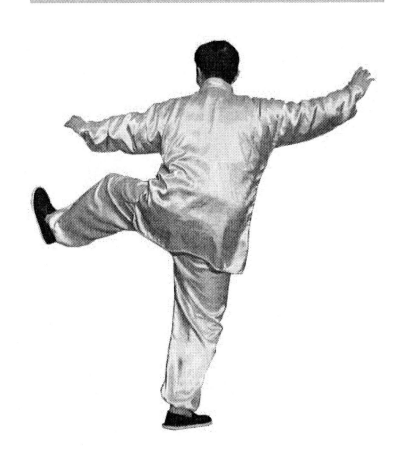

## Sequence of Form 15 —Turn and Kick with Left Heel

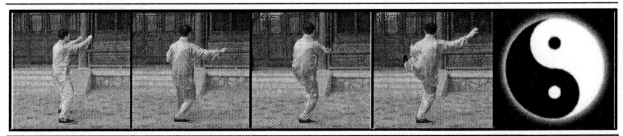

We push downward then up on the left leg.  Some call this "Left Golden Cock."

[16a]: left leg steps out left and left arm moves down and forward inside the left leg;

[16b]: right arm back, right hand held in hook;

[16c]: right knee rises, right hand held high.

## Group 5

### Form 16: Left Down One-leg Stand

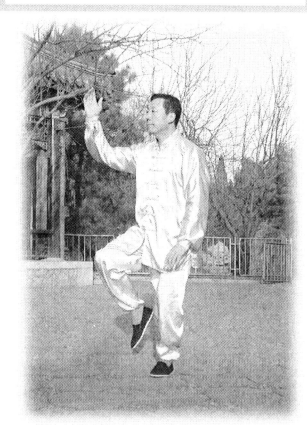

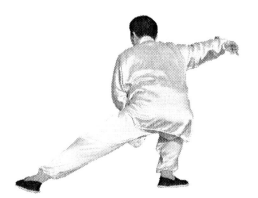

## Sequence of Form 16 —Left Down One-leg Stand

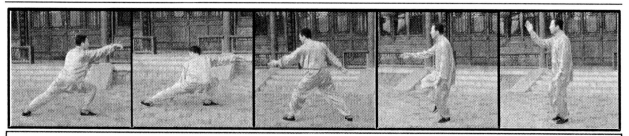

# Tai Chi for Health

In Form 17, first push downward then stand on right leg (or called Right Golden Cock).

**Form 17: Right Down One-leg Stand**

[17a]: right leg steps out right and right arm moves down and forward inside the right leg;

[17b]: right arm back, right hand held in hook;

[17c]: left knee raises, left hand held high.

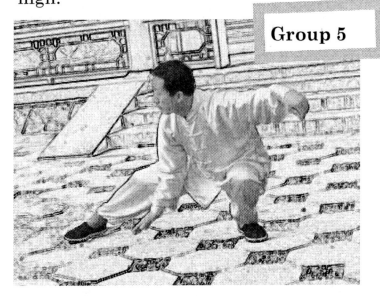

**Group 5**

## Sequence of Form 17 —Right Down One-leg Stand

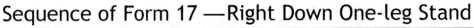

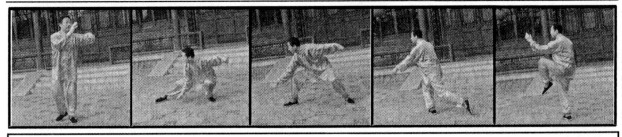

**Group 5**

Form 18: Work at Shuttles

Some calls Form 18 "Fair Lady Works at Shuttles. This is another push form that consists of both left and right side moves.

[18a]: Right Side: right arm blocks upward, left palm strikes forward;

[18b]: Left Side: left arm blocks upward, right palm strikes forward.

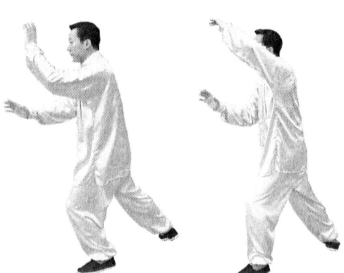

## Sequence of Form 18 —Name of the form

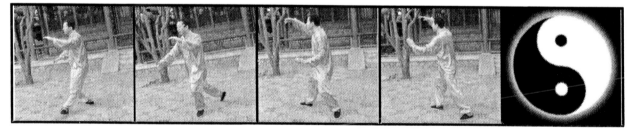

## Sequence of Form 18 Continued

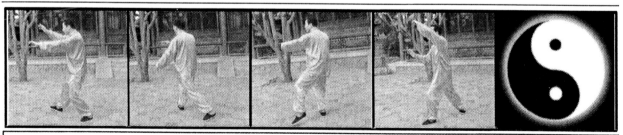

## Group 5

### Form 19: Find a Needle at Sea Bottom

We shift balance backward , bow down and reach out the right hand like searching an object. Indeed, Form 19 looks like someone finding a needle at the bottom of the sea.

[19a]: sit on the right leg;

[19b]: point down with left hand.

## Sequence of Form 19 —Find a Needle at Sea Bottom

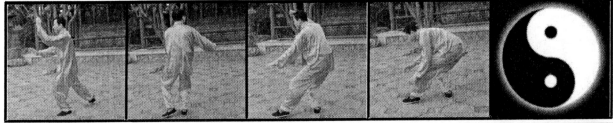

**Group 5**

**Form 20: Flash Arms**

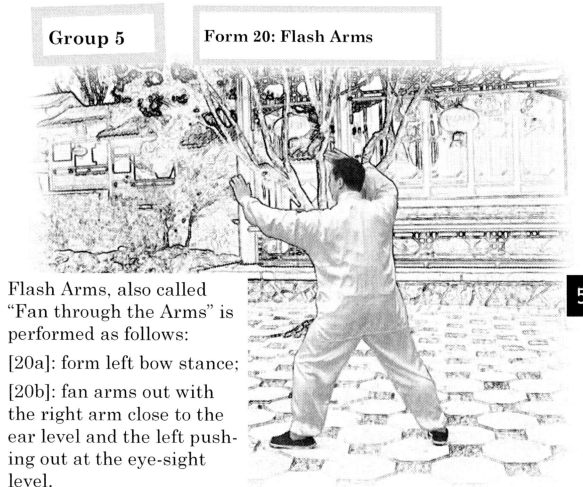

Flash Arms, also called "Fan through the Arms" is performed as follows:

[20a]: form left bow stance;

[20b]: fan arms out with the right arm close to the ear level and the left pushing out at the eye-sight level.

53

## Sequence of Form 20 —Flash Arms

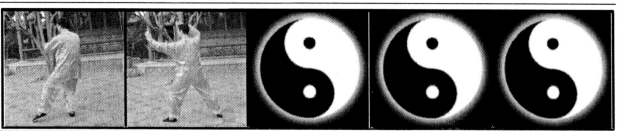

# Tai Chi for Health

## Group 6

### Form 21: Turn to Deflect, Block, and Strike

Form 21 is a sequence of turn, deflect
downward, parry, and punch.

**54**

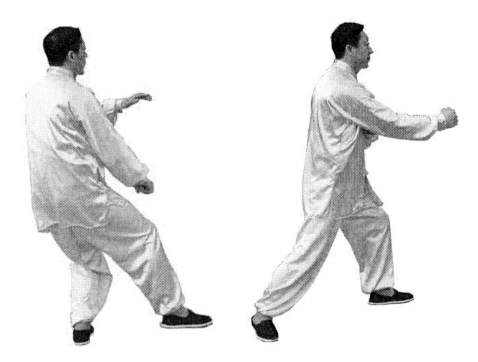

## Sequence of Form 21 —Turn to Deflect, Block, and Strike

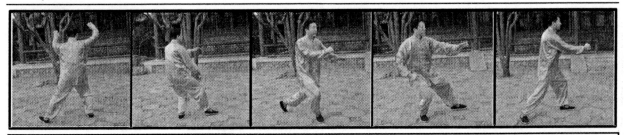

## Group 6

### Form 22: Seal as Close-up

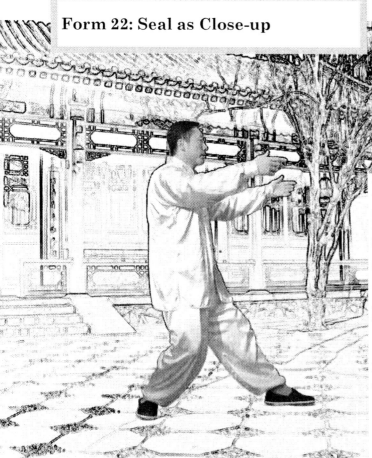

Form 22: Close up.

[22a]: Left hand moves under right arm, draw both arms back;

[22b]: Shift 80% of weight back to the right leg;

[22c]: Shift center forward in a left bow stance, push with two hands.

## Sequence of Form 22 —Seal as Close-up

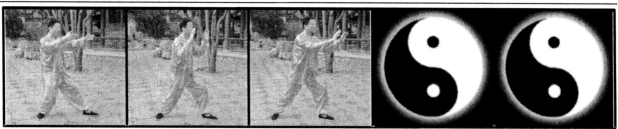

# Tai Chi for Health

## Group 6

## Form 23: Cross Hands

Form 23 forms a posture of crossing hands at the chest level.

[23a]: both feet open shoulder width apart, weight distributed on both legs evenly;

[23b]: Hands crossed at chest, right hand in front.

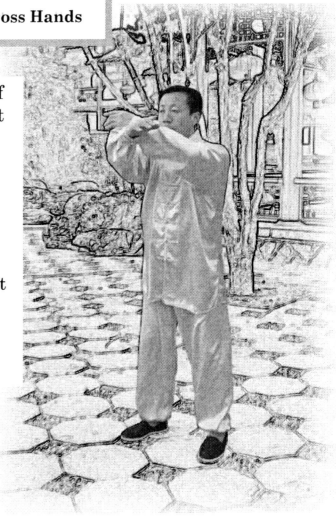

## Sequence of Form 23 —Cross Hands

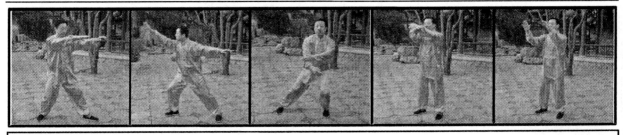

**Group 6**　　**Form 24: Conclusion**

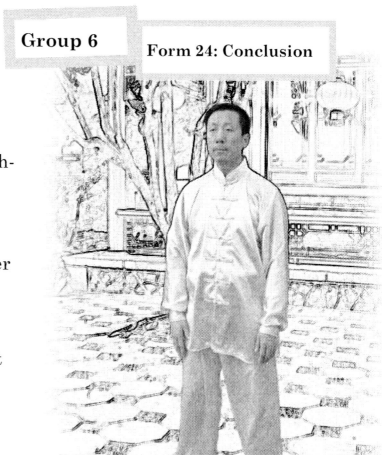

Form 24 is the finishing form.

[24a]:  raise both hands up to shoulder level then lower to waist;

[24b]: move the left foot beside the right foot.

## Sequence of Form 24 —Conclusion

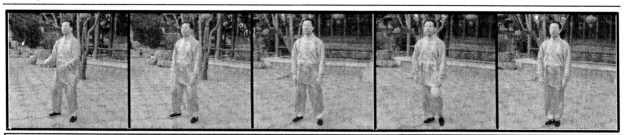

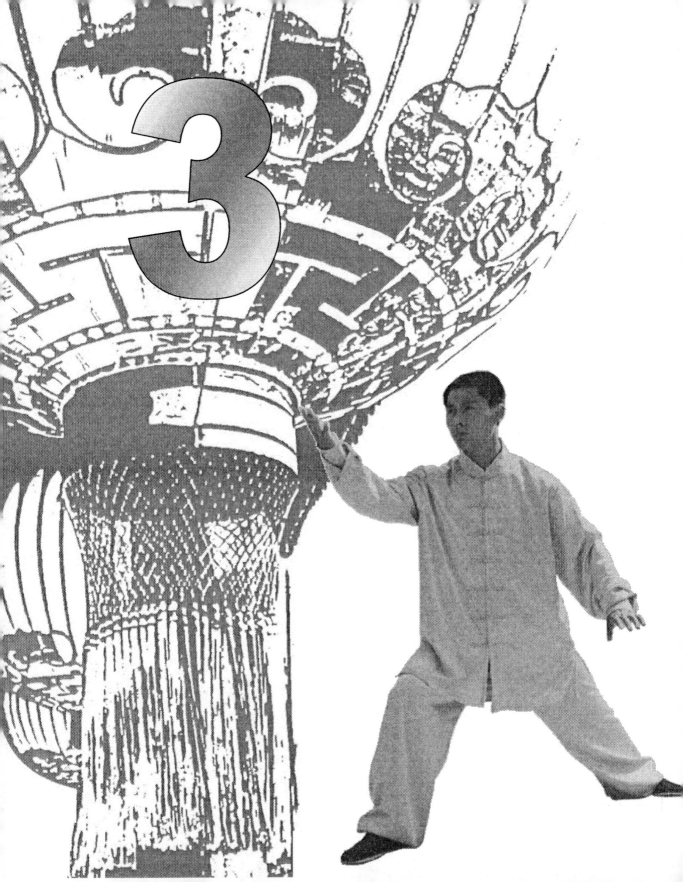

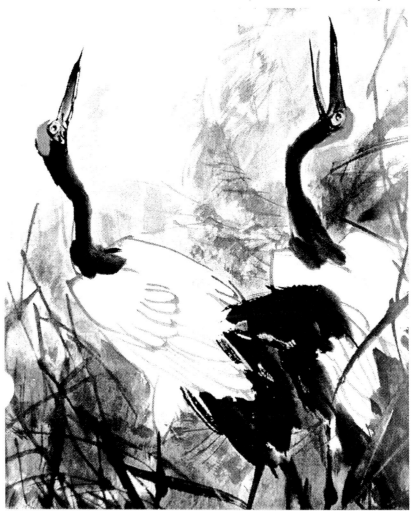

## Tai Chi has its principles

In order to learn Tai Chi successfully, you will need to have a good level of understanding of the principles that were passed down over the centuries by Tai Chi masters. These principles are presented here with great simplification but shall be the foundation of Tai Chi and used as guidelines for those who are learning and practicing the art.

# Tai Chi for Health

A Tai Chi practitioner shall be consistent with the way he or she stands, looks and moves. These are the key to the smooth transitions that convey Tai Chi moves. Here, the principles of Tai Chi Posture are explained in the order of head, neck, chest, shoulder, elbow, wrist, waist, hip, knee, leg, ankle, and foot.

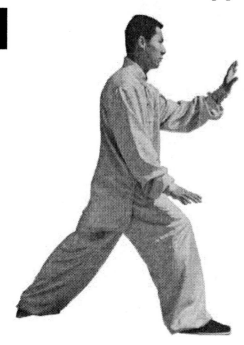

[1]  Head upright with spirit of lightness;

[2]  Neck relaxed and upright;

[3]  Chest in with back raised;

[4]  Shoulders sunk naturally;

[5]  Elbows dropped as they go;

[6]  Hands naturally extended;

[7]  Wrist naturally curved up;

[8]  Waist and limb relaxed;

[9]  Hip relaxed backward;

[10]  Knees bent and stretched coordinately;

[11]  Legs balanced with any size of steps;

[12]  Ankles support solid steps;

[13]  Foot flat on the group.

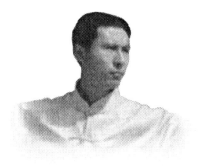

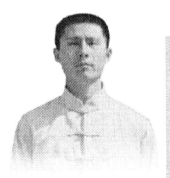

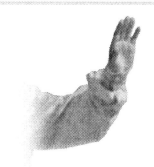

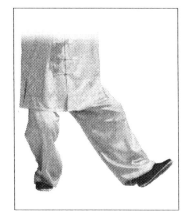

**Posture of head, neck and shoulders**

**Waist and hip**

**Posture of hand and wrist**

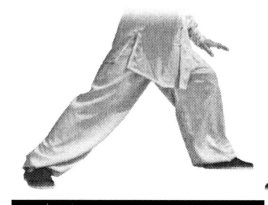

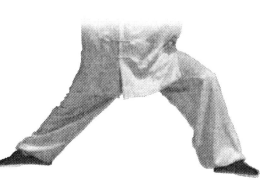

**Legs, knees, and feet**

**Legs, knees, ankles and feet**

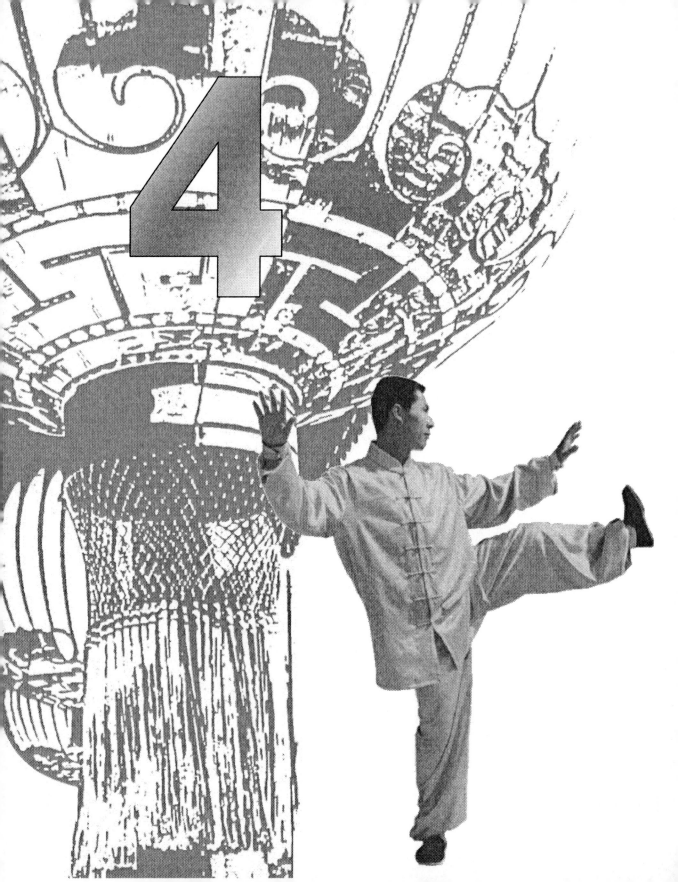

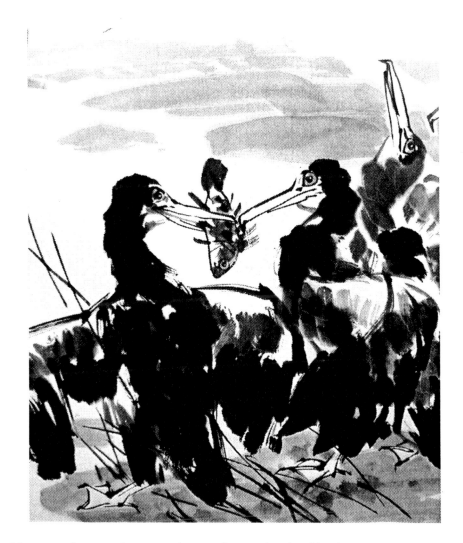

63

## Keep the orientations in mind all the time

The actions of feet should be light but firm. Further-more, the orientation of steps determines the next move. Good orientations makes connecting moves smooth.

In the practice of Tai Chi, there exists a long history of movement theory and exercise systems that are associated with Taoism or Feng Shui.  In some sense, the elements of Taoism and Feng Shui are the contributing  factors to what directions a person shall face or how a body move should be performed.  By Chinese tradition, a Tai Chi person shall face south (where the light comes from) at the Starting Form and the closing form.  In the following, a sequence chart is used to show the body directions in each group of Tai Chi moves.  A compass is used for the reference of direction.  Notice here the compass is drawn upside down for the ease of associating the body position of reading to that of  Tai Chi practicing ; the upside points to south, not north.  A parallelogram is used with the long side representing the front of a person and the short side for the back of the person.

**64**

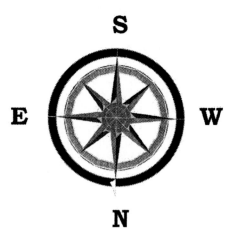

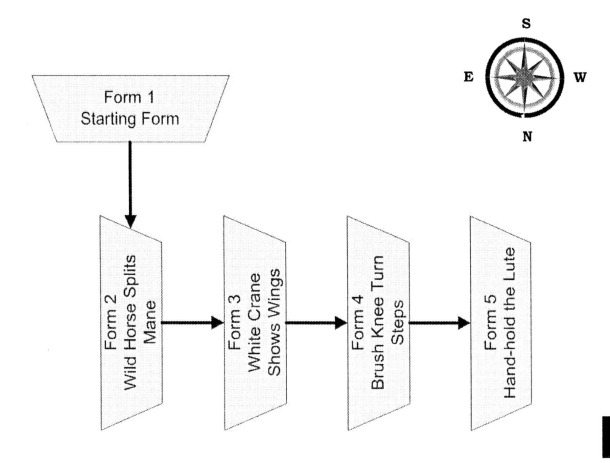

To start Form 1, stand facing south.  It is advised to do some
warm-up exercise before start.  A little warm-up will help relax
the body and ankles and reduce the risk of injury even though
Tai Chi is a slowing moving workout.  As your body turns to the
left when you start From 2, you start to face south shown by
the long side of the parallelogram.  In the following three forms
(Form 3—5), you keep the same direction as in Form 2.

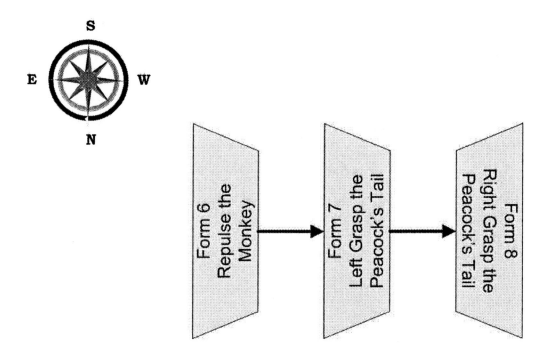

66

After Form 5 (Hand-hold the Lute), you take you step back for Form 6 (Repulse the Monkey). At this point, you still face east as the long side of the parallelogram shown above. You may have small body turns in Form 7, but you mainly face east until the end of From 7. You perform a 180 degree turn to transition from Form 7 to Form 8. Now you face west as the long side of parallelogram shown above. Note the turn of your body should be well coordinated with the turn and the slide of your steps to make the transition smooth and steady.

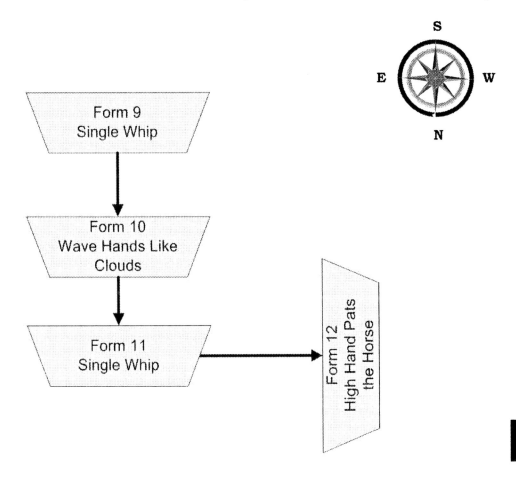

When Starting Form 9, you come back to face south as you are in the beginning form (Form 1).  The Single Whip is a short time posture in which your body faces south but you look at your left hand with your shoulder slightly turned to East.  You slide your steps to the left in Form 10, but still face south.  Form 10 is connected with the Single Whip again.  Now you turn your body to east to perform Form 12.

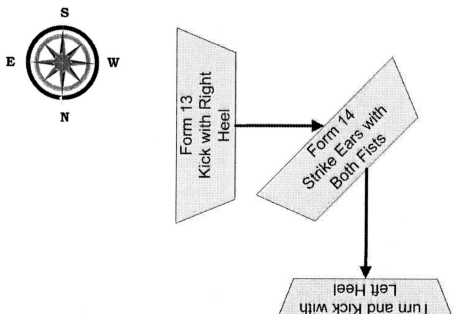

**68**

In form 13, you keep facing east.  The strike with both fists in Form 14 turns your body 45 degrees to face southeast.  Then a wide turn takes you to face north.  Now you are in Form 15. After you do left-down in Form 16, you stand up with one leg facing west.  The following chart shows this direction for Form 16.  You mainly face west from Form 16 throughout Form 20.  A complete 180 degree turn is made to transition from Form 20 to Form 21 (the turn part of Form 21).  Then, you do deflect, block and strike.  At the end of Form 22, you slide your right foot to west and turn your body to face south again to do  Cross Hands (Form 23).  Take your hands down and right foot back and now you come the conclusion form to finish the entire 24 forms.

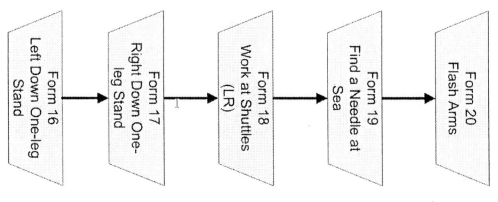

Form 16
Left Down One-leg Stand → Form 17
Right Down One-leg Stand → Form 18
Work at Shuttles (LR) → Form 19
Find a Needle at Sea → Form 20
Flash Arms

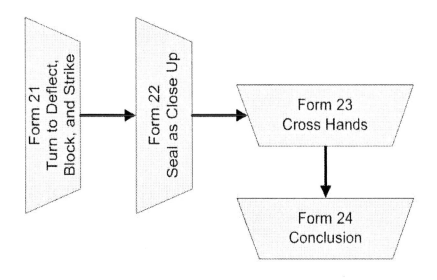

Form 21
Turn to Deflect, Block, and Strike → Form 22
Seal as Close Up → Form 23
Cross Hands → Form 24
Conclusion

69

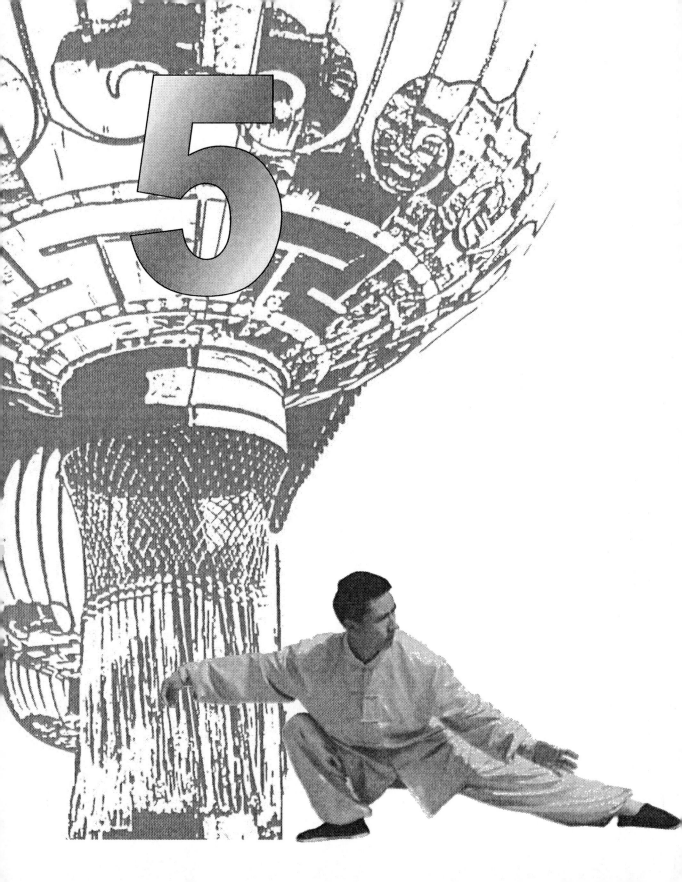

# Orientation and Positions

*East*
*South*
*West*
*North*

In performing these 24 forms, you should imagine you are standing in the middle of a compass. You are facing south, directly behind you is north. To your right is west and to your left is east. Southwest is halfway between south and west. Southeast is halfway between south and east. Northwest is halfway between north and west. And northeast is halfway between north and east. Although your position will change as you move through the Forms, these directions will remain fixed. Keeping these directions in your mind will help with the orientation of your body and steps in practice and master Tai Chi moves quickly.

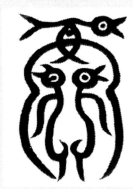

71

**Group One**

*Form 1: Starting Form*

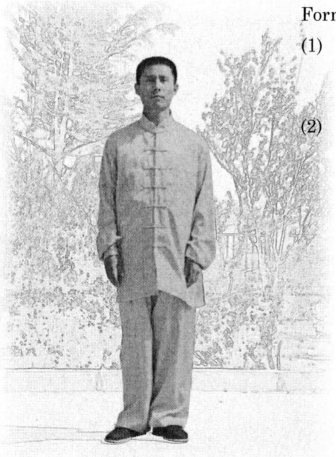

Form 1: Starting Form.

(1) Stand relaxed with both feet close, facing south. Breathe naturally.

(2) Shift your body weight to the right leg; lift the left foot softly and move it about one's shoulder width to the left. Center the body's weight evenly between both legs. Breath should be regulated and even. While lifting the left foot, inhale; when placing the foot down, exhale.

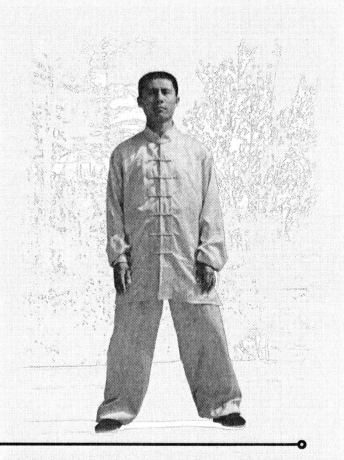

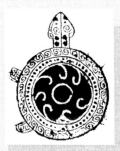

**Starting from South**

Points to follow: allow your arms to hang at your sides naturally, keep your neck and back straight and upright. The chin is slightly tucked in, your eyes gaze forward with concentrated spirit. The chest is sunken, the back is arced and the shoulders rounded. Keep your body centered and upright.  Relax your whole body.

Try your best to just enjoy the moment. Relax and sink into a state of consciousness that can be characterized as calm, peaceful, open, joyful, content, unhurried, and uplifting. If worries, concerns, memories, daydreams, joys, or thoughts come into your mind, then just note them and allow them to pass away. Be aware of the energy within your body.

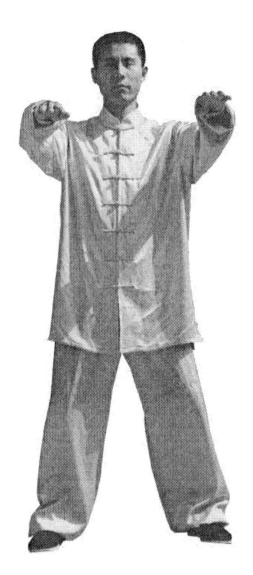

(3)    Slowly raise both arms to shoulder height. Arms are kept parallel to each other with the palms facing down. When the arms reach shoulder level, then lower both arms pressing the palm down gently to the waist. Allow both knees to bend slightly into a comfortable position.

Points to follow: Hold your head and neck erect, with the chin slightly drawn in. Do not stand erect with the chest protruding and the abdomen drawn in. Keep torso erect and relaxed with the shoulders rounded. Elbows are down and the fingers are slightly curved. Body weight is equally distributed between legs. While bending knees, keep the waist relaxed and buttocks slightly tucked in.

As you raise your hands, breathe in. As you lower your hands, breathe out. Breathe from the abdomen. Allow your abdomen (belly) to relax outward as you breathe in. As you breathe out, gently suck your abdomen inward to force the air out of your lungs.

# Chapter 5  Detailed Description

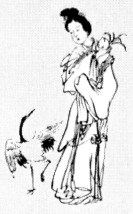

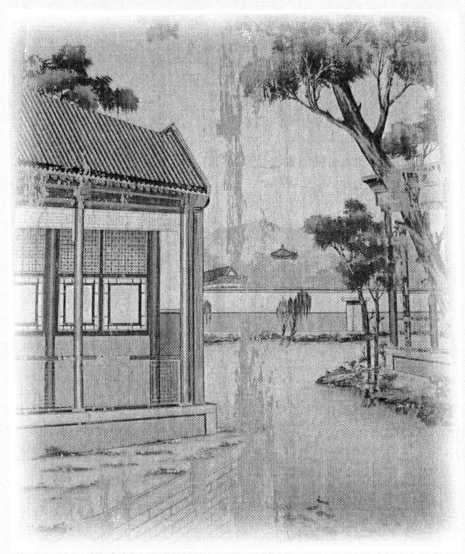

**Group One**

*Form 2: Wild Horse Splits Mane*

(1) Shift the weight to the right leg and move the left foot close to the right foot while turning the body slightly to the left. At the same time, move both hands and arms to the front as if holding a large ball. Look at the right hand. Face south.

76

(2) Step out with the left foot into a left Bow stance. As you settle into the left Bow stance, place the left heel down first and allow the foot to roll forward. Seventy percent of your weight should now be on the left leg. While making this movement, the left arm curves upward to shoulder level with the left hand held forward and at eye level. The right arms curves down with right palm down to guard the right waist. The eye follows the left hand. The body is now facing southeast.

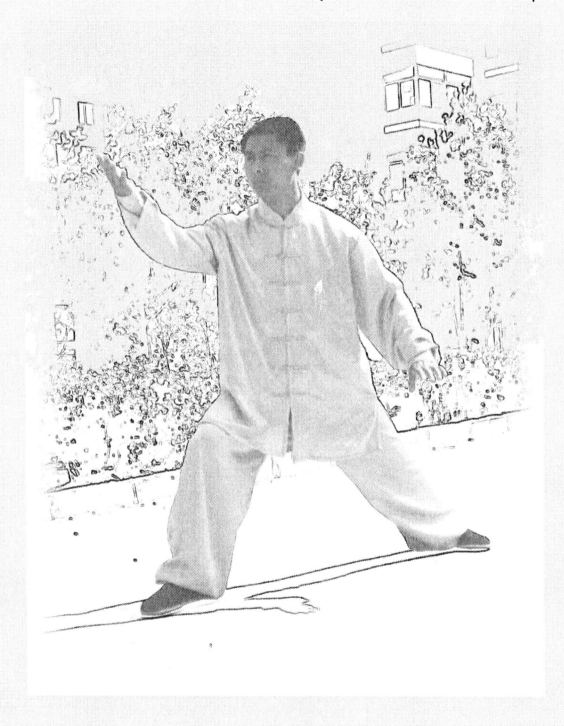

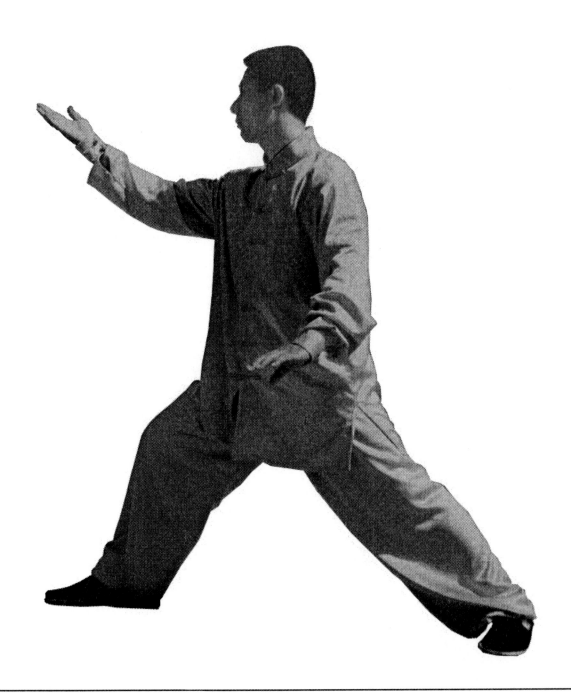

(3) Shift your weight backward onto the right leg. Pivot on the left heel and allow the left foot to move outward 45 degrees. Shift the body gently forward onto the left leg. Draw the right foot forward placing it near the left foot with the toe touching the floor. At the same time, both arms and hands move to the left as if holding a large ball. You are now facing north with eyes focused on the left hand.

(4) Step out with the right foot into a right Bow stance. As you settle into the right Bow stance, place the right heel down first and allow the foot to roll forward. Seventy percent of your weight should now be on the right leg. While making this movement, the right arm curves upward to shoulder level with the right hand held forward and at eye level. The left arms curves down with left palm down to guard the left waist. The eye follows the right hand. The body is now facing northeast

(5) Shift your weight backward onto the left leg. Pivot on the right heel and allow the right foot to move outward 45 degrees. Shift the body gently forward onto the right leg. Draw the left foot forward placing it near the left foot with the toe touching the floor. At the same time, both arms and hands move to the right as if holding a large ball. You are now facing south with eyes focused on the right hand.

79

**Beast Bites Back**

(6) Step out with the left foot into a left Bow stance. As you settle into the left Bow stance, place the left heel down first and allow the foot to roll forward. Seventy percent of your weight should now be on the left leg. While making this movement, the left arm curves upward to shoulder level with the left hand held forward and at eye level. The right arms curves down with right palm down to guard the right waist. The eye follows the left hand. The body is now facing southeast.

Points to follow: Hold the torso erect and keep the chest relaxed. Sink the arms and drop the elbows. Move arms in a curve when you separate hands. Relax the waist. Use waist as the axis in body turns. The movements in taking a bow stance and separating hands must be smooth and synchronized. When taking a bow stance, place the front foot slowly into position with the heel coming down first. The knee of front leg should not extend beyond toes of the front foot. There should be a transverse distance of 10-30cm between heels.

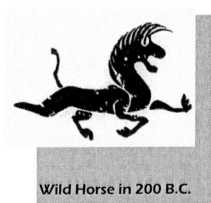

**Wild Horse in 200 B.C.**

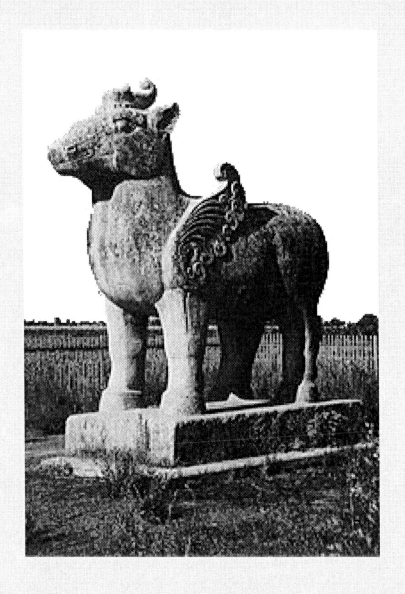

## Group One

### *Form 3: White Crane Shows Wings*

Form 3 is also called "White Crane Spreads Its Wings" in some books. A more literal translation is used here.

(1) Shift the body center onto the left leg. Lift the right foot half step forward, placing it behind the left leg. Lightly shift the body center backward to sit on the right leg. Extend the left toe a little forward into an empty stance. At the same time, both arms and hands form a circle, as if holding a large ball, the left hand above the right hand. Face east.

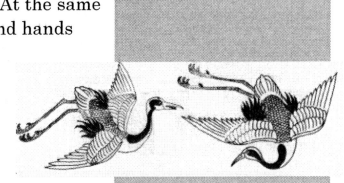

**White Cranes Show Their Wings**

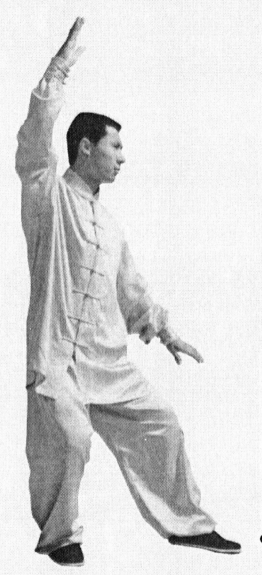

(2) Rotate the body to the right slightly. Lift the right arm upward and with the right hand pointing ups above the head. Move the left arm and hand down to guard the left waist.

Points to remember: Do not thrust the chest forward. Arms should be rounded when they move up and down. Left knee is slightly curved. Eighty percent of your weight sits on the right leg.

83

## Group One

### *Form 4: Brush Knee Turn Steps*

Form 4 goes as if we brush knee on one side with a twist step first and the push hand on the other side. This form repeats three times from left to right and to left again.

(1) Rotate the waist slightly to the left and then back to the right. The right arm circles down across the face with the palm facing inward. Continue moving the right hand down past the navel; then circling upward with the palm at ear level. Move the left hand up in a circular motion past the face with the left palm coming to guard the right

**84**

elbow. At the same time, lift the left foot and bring it close to the right foot. Look at the right hand. You are facing south-east.

(2) Rotate the waist to the left and step out with the left foot placing the left heel on the floor first. Move 70% of your body weight forward to the front left leg and come to rest in a left bow stance. Left hand moves downward as if brushing the

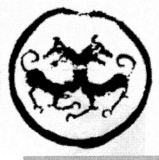

**Pushing Forces Turning**

left knee while the right palm pushes forward. You now face east.

(3) Shift your weight backward onto the right leg. Pivot on the left heel and allow the left foot to move outward 45 degrees. Shift the body gently forward onto the left leg. Draw the right foot forward placing it near the left foot with the toe touching the floor. At the same time, bend the right arm and move the right hand before the face. Circle the left arm outward and back and then to the front across the face. Look at the left hand and face northeast.

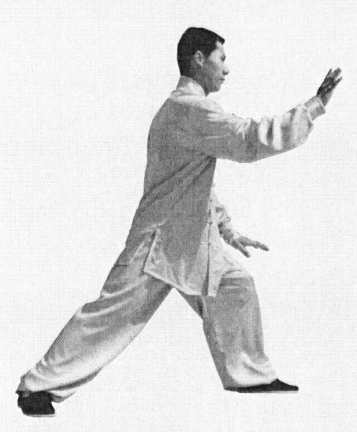

(4) Rotate the waist to the left and step out with the right foot placing the left heel on the floor first. Move 70% of your body weight forward to the right leg and come to rest in a right bow stance. Right hand moves downward as if brushing the right knee while the left palm pushes forward. You now face east.

85

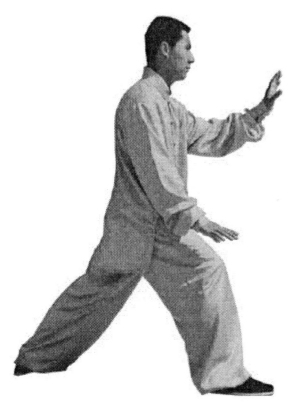

(5) Shift your weight backward onto the left leg. Pivot on the right heel and allow the right foot to move outward 45 degrees. Shift the body gently forward onto the right leg. Draw the left foot forward placing it near the right foot with the toe touching the floor. At the same time, bend the left arm and move the left hand before the face. Circle the right arm outward and back and then to the front across the face. Look at the right hand. You face southeast.

(6) Rotate the waist to the left and step out with the left foot placing the left heel on the floor first. Move 70% of your body weight forward onto the left leg and come to rest in a left bow stance. Left hand moves downward as if brushing the left knee while the right palm pushes forward. You now face east.

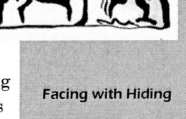

**Facing with Hiding**

Points to follow: Keep torso erect while pushing palm forward. Sink shoulders and elbow down while pushing palm forward. Relax the waist. The movements of the palm should be coordinated with those of waist and legs. Move arms in a curve. Use waist as the axis in body turns. The movements in taking a bow stance and brushing/pushing hands must be smooth and synchronized in tempo. When taking a bow stance, place front foot slowly in position, heel coming down first. The knee of front leg should not go beyond toes. Keep a transverse distance of 30cm between heels in bow stance.

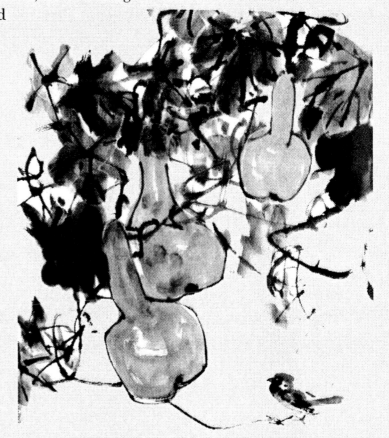

**Group One**

*Form 5: Hand-hold the Lute*

Form 5 resembles a person playing a lute, a common music instrument in old China's time. It is more accurate to describe it as hands holding the lute, which is also a literal translation from its counterpart in Chinese.

(1) Shift the body weight onto the left leg. Lift the right foot and move it half step forward, placing it behind the left foot.

(2) Lightly shift the body center back to sit on the right leg. Extend the left heel a little forward touching the floor in an empty stance. At the same time, rotate the waist slightly to the right, lift the left arm and hand upward to the nose level, lower the right hand to guard the inside of the left elbow. Face east.

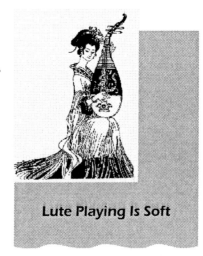

**Lute Playing Is Soft**

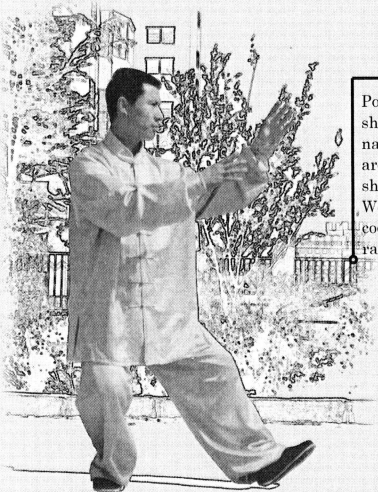

Points to follow: Steps should be steady and natural.  Relax the chest, arc the back, and sink shoulders and elbows.  Weight transfer must be coordinated with the raising of left hand.

89

Points to follow: Keep torso erect and shoulders and elbow down with enough space under arm for holding a chicken egg.  Shift the weight to the rear leg and look forward.  Do not open arms and elbows too wide or too high.

# Tai Chi for Health

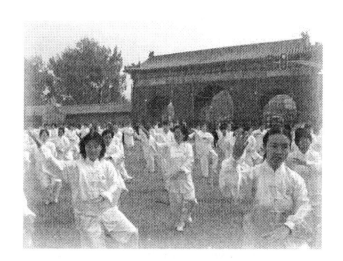
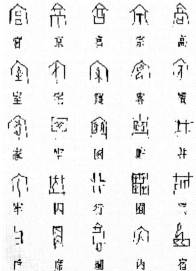

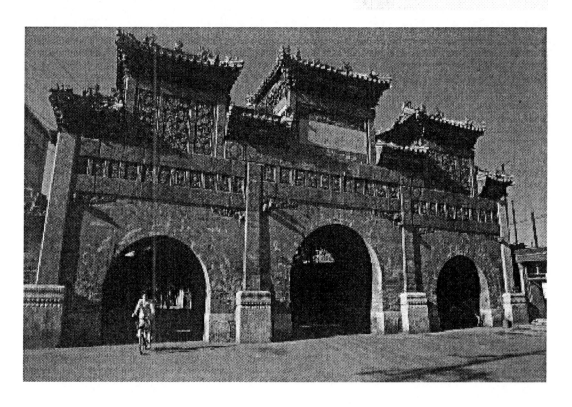

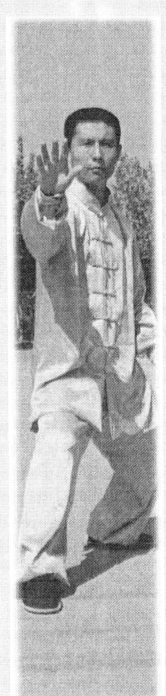

Group two consists of three
forms, each of which contains
a combination of moves.
Grasp the Peacock's Tail is
the largest form in all 24
forms in terms of the moves
contained in this form.

| Group 2 | |
| --- | --- |
| 6. Repulse the Monkey | 92 |
| 7. Left Grasp the Peacock's Tail | 96 |
| 8. Right Grasp the Peacock's Tail | 100 |

# Tai Chi for Health

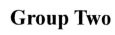

**Group Two**

*Form 6: Repulse the Monkey*

Step back first and then whirl arms as if we were repulsing a monkey. Perform this move four times: left, right, left, and right.

(1) Rotate your body center to the right and pull the right hand downward, back, and up in a semicircle to shoulder level. The right arm and hand are extended backward with the right

**92**

palm up. The left arm is extended forward with the palm up. The body is centered on and sits on the right leg. Look at the right hand.

(2) Bring the right hand toward the right ear and rotate the body center to the left. Push the right hand forward and pull the left hand down beside the waist with the left palm up. At the same time, lift the left foot and step back to sit on the left leg. Look at the right hand.

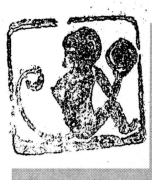

**Happy with Peach**

(3) Rotate your body center to the left and pull the left hand downward, back, and up in a semicircle to shoulder level. The left arm and hand are extended backward with the left palm up. The right arm is extended forward with the palm up. The body is centered on and sits on the left leg. Look at the left hand.

(4) Bring the left hand toward the left ear and rotate the body center to the right. Push the left hand forward and pull the right hand down beside the waist with the right palm up. At the same time, lift the right foot and step back to sit on the right leg position. Look at the left hand.

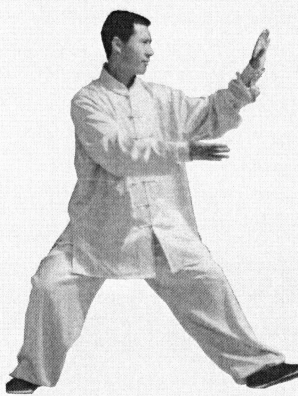

93

(5) Rotate your body center to the right and pull the right hand downward, back, and up in a semicircle to shoulder level. The right arm and hand are extended backward with the right palm up. The left arm is extended forward with the palm up. The body is centered on and sits on the right leg. Look at the right hand.

(6) Bring the right hand toward the right ear and rotate the body center to the left. Push the right hand forward and pull the left hand down beside the waist with the left palm up. As the same time, lift the left foot and step back to sit on the left leg. Look at the right hand.

(7) Rotate your body center to the left and pull the left hand downward, back, and up in a semicircle to shoulder level. The left arm and hand are extended backward with the left palm up. The right arm is extended forward with the palm up. The body is centered on and sits on the left leg. Look at the left hand.

(8) Bring the left hand toward the left ear and rotate the body center to the right. Push the left hand forward and pull the right hand down beside the waist with the right palm up. At the same time, lift the right foot and step back to sit on the right leg position. Look at the left hand.

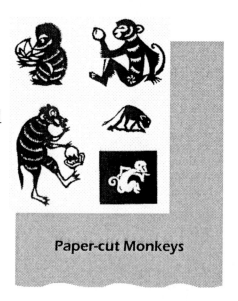

**Paper-cut Monkeys**

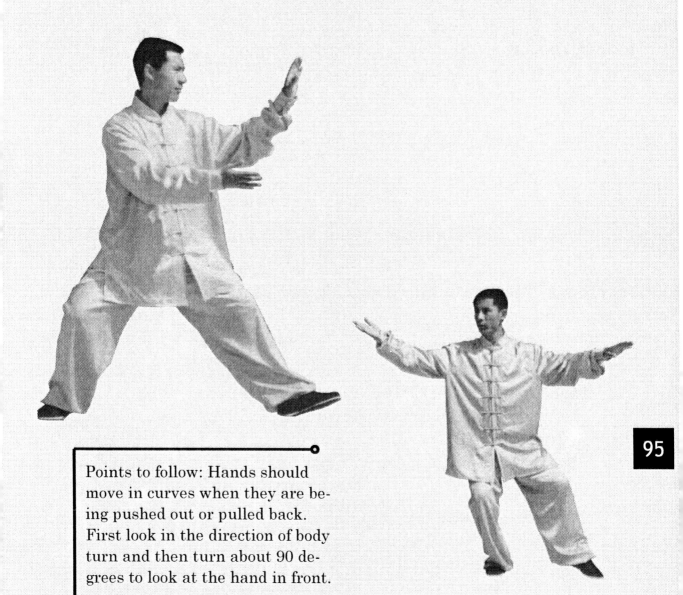

Points to follow: Hands should move in curves when they are being pushed out or pulled back. First look in the direction of body turn and then turn about 90 degrees to look at the hand in front.

**Group Two**

*Form 7: Left Grasp the Peacock's Tail*

Form 7: Grasp the Peacock's Tail (on the Left):

(1) Shift the body center to the right leg and rotate the waist to the south while both arms hold a large ball with the right hand above the left hand. Face the south.

(2) Ward off left: rotate your waist 90 degrees to the left and step forward with your left foot into a left bow stance. Your heel should touch down first.  As you settle into the bow stance, your left arm moves up so the left palm faces your chest. The right hand presses downward to guard the waist.  You now face the east. Gently, arc both hands slightly to the left. The left palm faces down and the right palm faces up.

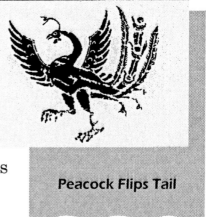

**Peacock Flips Tail**

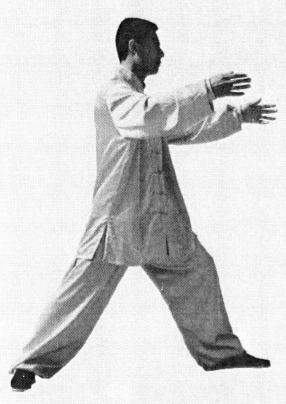

Points to follow: Keep both arms rounded and circular while moving them. The separation of hands, turning of waist and bending of leg should be coordinated.

(3) Roll Back: Rotate your waist 45 degrees to the left. Allow your arms to follow the rotation of your body. While you rotate to the left, keep both palms the same relative positions in such that the left palm is down and the right palm is up. Rotate your body to the right so you are sitting on your right leg. At the same time, swing both arms backward following the pull of gravity until they are level with the right shoulder and you are looking at the right palm. Rotate back toward the east, placing the right hand close to the left wrist in front of your chest. Body center is still sitting on the right leg.

Points to follow: While pulling hands down, do not lean forward or let the buttocks protrude. Arms should follow the turning of waist and move in a circular path.

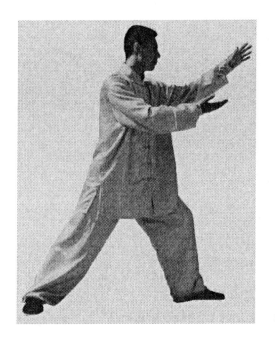

Points to follow: The movements of hands should be coordinated with the turning of waist and bending of the front leg.

Points to follow: Keep torso erect while pressing hands forward.

(4) Press: Move the body center forward into a left bow stance while pressing the left arm using the right palm. You now face east.

98

(5) Push: Sit back on the right leg while pulling both arms back so hands are near the waist level. Push the arms back up to shoulder level while pushing forward into a left bow stance. You now face east.

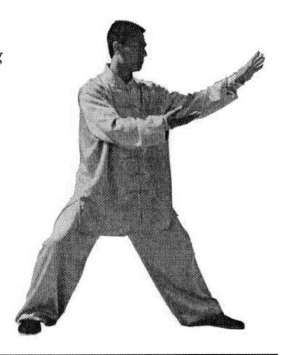

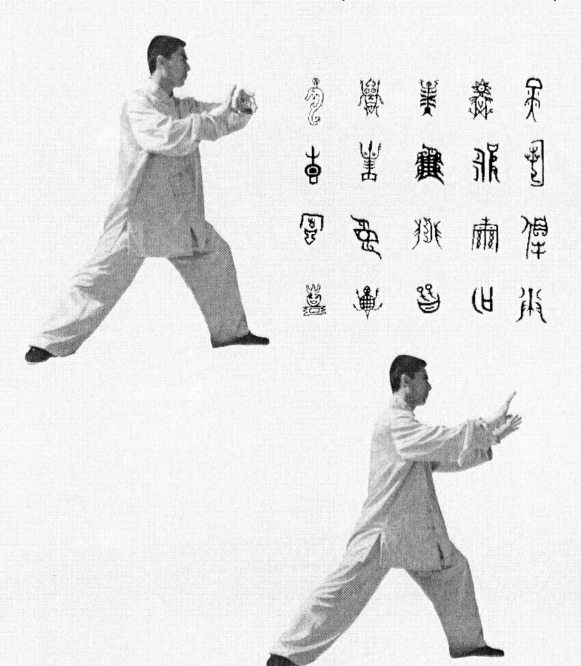

**Group Two**

## *Form 8: Right Grasp the Peacock's Tail*

Form 8: Grasp the Peacock's Tail (on the Right):

(1) While holding your arms extended, shift your weight to the right leg. Turn the left foot on the heel to the right. Move your waist to the right with your arms following the turning of your body. Draw back the right foot back so the toe rests beside the left foot. At the same time,

move your arms apart so the right palm is underneath the left palm as if holding a large ball. You face south.

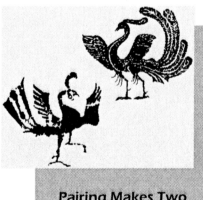

**Pairing Makes Two**

(2) Ward off right: rotate your waist 90 degrees to the right and step forward with your right foot into a right bow stance. Your heel should touch down first. As you settle into the bow stance, your right arm moves up so

the right palm faces your chest. The left hand presses downward to guard the waist.  You now face the west.

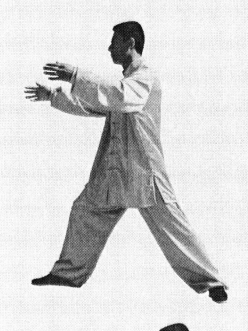

Gently, arc both hands slightly to the right. The right palm faces down and the left palm faces up.

(3) Roll Back: Rotate your waist 45 degrees to the right. Allow your arms to follow the rotation of your body. While you rotate to the right, keep both palms the same shape and relative positions so the right  palm is down and the left palm is up. Rotate your body to the left so you are sitting on your left leg. At the same time, swing both arms backward following the pull of gravity until they are level with the left shoulder and you are looking at the left palm. Rotate back toward the west, placing the left hand close to the right wrist in front of your chest. Body center is still sitting on the left leg.

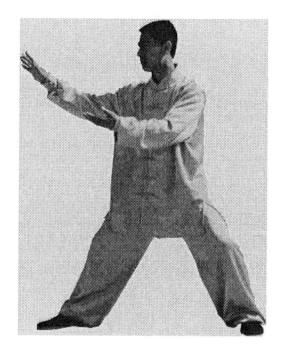

(4) Press: Move the body center forward into a right bow stance while pressing the right arm using the left palm. You now face west.

(5) Push: Sit back on the left leg while pulling both arms back so hands are near the waist level. Push the arms back up to shoulder level while pushing forward into a left bow stance. You now face west.

# Chapter 5  Detailed Description

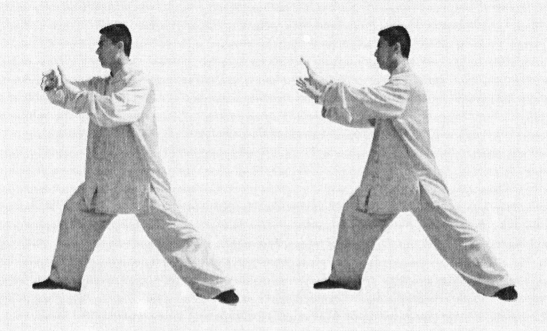

## Group Three

### *Form 9: Single Whip*

Form 9: Single Whip.

(1) Sit back and pivot to the left on the right heel with the toe turning inward. Both arms are extended outward at shoulder level and describe a half circle as you turn. Shift your center to the right leg. At the same time, form the right hand

into a hook with the fingers and thumb joined together and pointed down. Your eyes look at the hook hand.

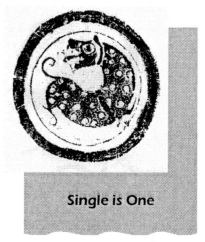

(2) Lift your left foot and place it forward in a left bow stance. At the same time, extend your left arm and push your palm forward. Look at the left hand. Face east.

**Single is One**

Points to follow: Keep torso erect, relax waist, and sink shoulders. Left palm is turned outward slowly, not too abruptly, as hand pushes forward. All transitional movements must be well coordinated.

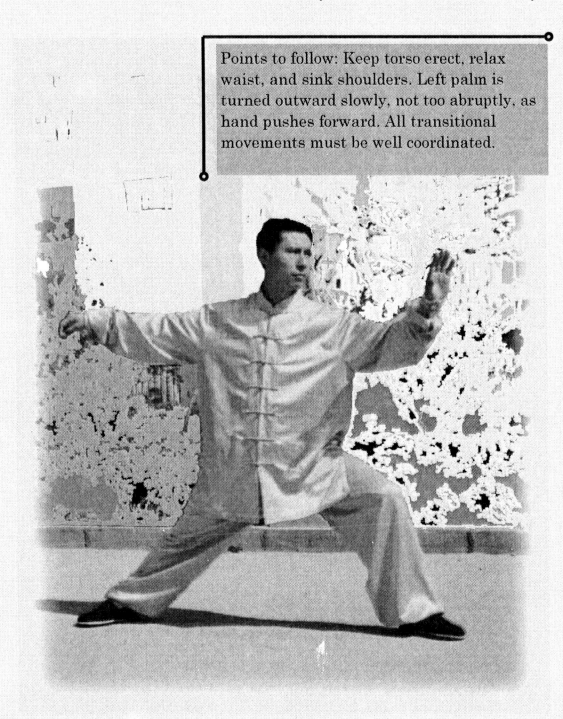

## Group Three

### Form 10: Wave Hands Like Clouds

Form 10: Wave Hands Like Clouds (1, 2, 3).

(1) Shift your body weight onto the right leg while rotating the waist to the right and turning the left foot inward towards the south. Circle the left arm downward and then upward to the right and at shoulder level. The left palm

turns up and the right palm faces down. Look towards the southwest.

(2) Shift your weight onto the left leg. Wave the left hand to the left side in front of your face. Press the right hand down and then up to become level with the left shoulder. At the same time draw the right foot parallel to the left foot with about two fists separating them. Face the southeast. Your weight is on the left leg.

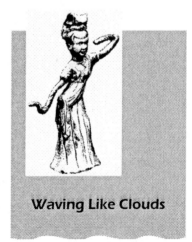

**Waving Like Clouds**

(3) Shift your weight to the right leg. Wave the right arm to the right, passing it in front of your face. Pull the left hand down, passing it in front of your lower waist and then upward to become level with the right shoulder.

(4) Lift your left foot and place it to the left parallel to the right foot. Shift your weight to the left leg. At the same time, wave the left hand to the left side in front of your face. Pull the right hand down and then up to become level with the left shoulder. At the same time draw the right foot parallel to the left foot with about two fists separating them. Face the southeast direction. Your center is on the left leg.

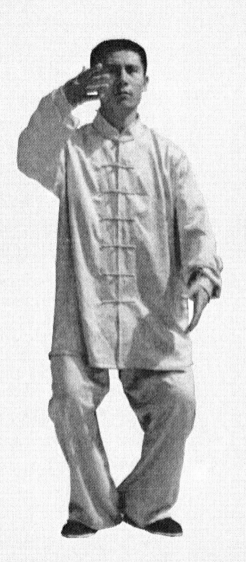

107

(5) Shift your weight to the right leg. Lift and wave the right hand to the right side in front of your face and pull the left hand down and then up to become level with the right shoulder.

(6) Lift your left foot and place it to the left parallel to the right foot. Shift your weight to the left leg. At the same time, wave the left hand to the left side in front of your face and pull the right hand down and then up to become level with the left shoulder. At the same time draw the right foot parallel to the left foot with about two fists separating them. Face the southeast. Your weight is centered on the left leg.

(7) Shift your weight to the right leg

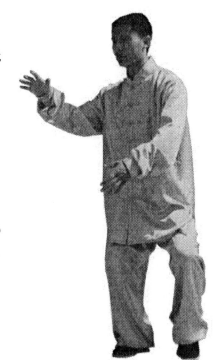

while rotating the waist to the right. Draw the left foot close to the right foot. Press the left hand down, passing it in front of your lower waist, and then up to become level with the right shoulder. At the same time, lift the right hand and wave it in front of face stopping level with the right shoulder. Form the right hand into a hook hand. Look to the southwest.

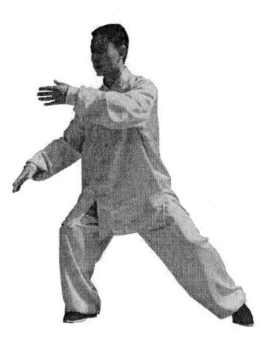

Points to follow: Use the spine as the axis when turning the body. Keep the waist and hip relaxed. Keep your body level; do not let the body rise and fall as you move. Arms are rounded. Arm movements should be natural and circular, following the movement of the waist. Pace must be slow and even. Arms and legs are coordinated. Both feet are parallel. Try to attain a good balance when moving the lower limbs. Your eyes should follow the hand as it moves in front of your face.

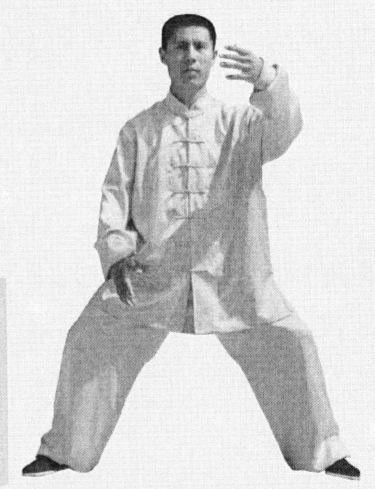

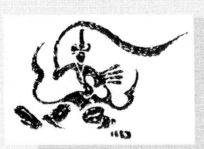

**Extending with Sleeves**

## Group Three

### Form 11: Single Whip

Repeat Form 9: Single Whip.

(1) Sit back and pivot to the left on the right heel with the toe turning inward. Both arms are extended outward at shoulder level and describe a half circle as you turn. Shift your center to the right leg. At the same time, form the right hand

into a hook with the fingers and thumb joined together and pointed down. Your eyes look at the hook hand.

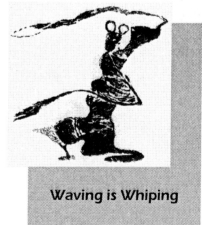

(2) Lift your left foot and place it forward in a left bow stance. At the same time, extend your left arm and push your palm forward. Look at the left hand. Face east.

**Waving is Whiping**

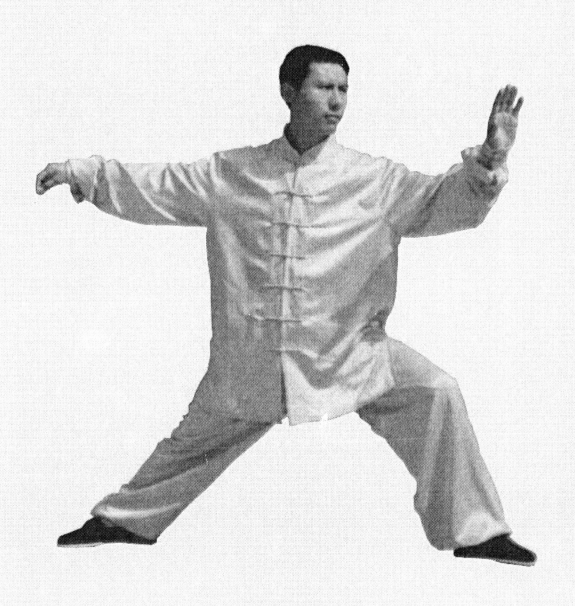

**Group Three**

*Form 12: High Hand Pats the Horse*

Form 12: High Pat the Horse.

(1) Shift your weight forward to the left leg, draw the right foot half a step forward behind the left leg, and then sit back on the right leg. At the same time, the hooked right hands comes open and both palms turn up.

(2) Rotate the body slightly left. Push the right palm forward past the right ear while pulling the left hand backward to rest beside the left side of the hip. Softly place the left foot forward with the toes touching the ground. Look at the east direction.

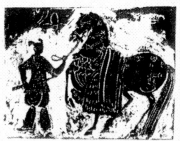

**Hand on Horse**

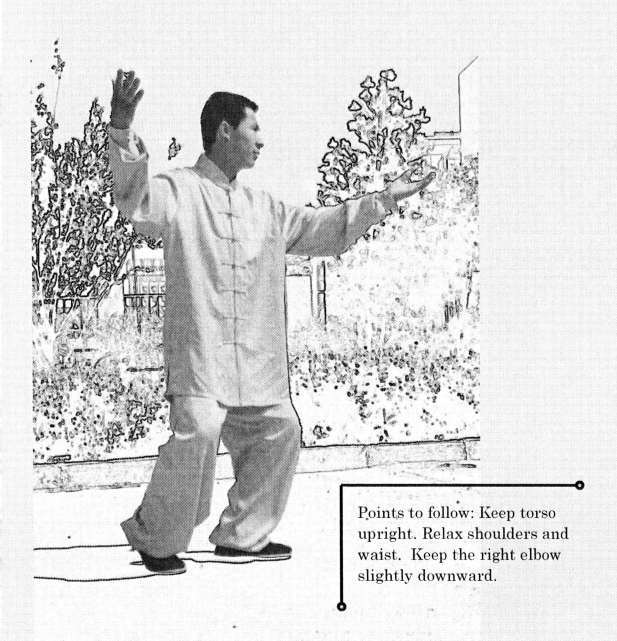

113

Points to follow: Keep torso upright. Relax shoulders and waist. Keep the right elbow slightly downward.

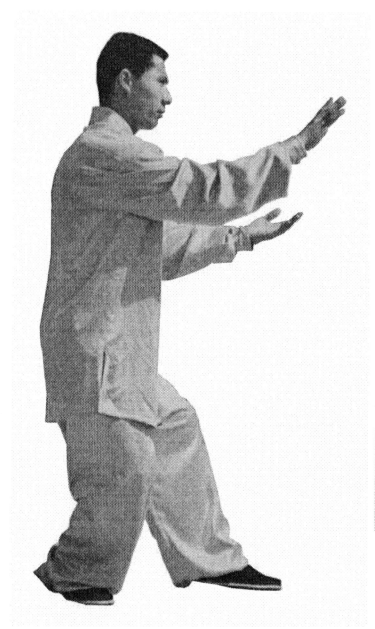

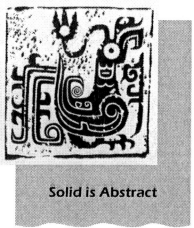

**Solid is Abstract**

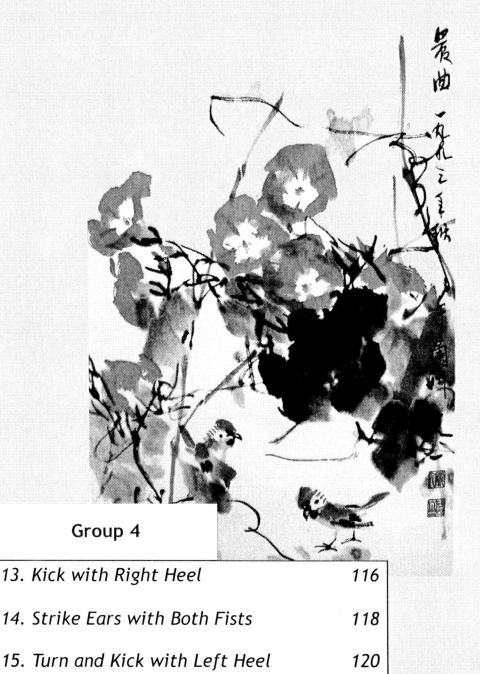

115

## Group 4

**Group Four**

*Form 13: Kick with Right Heel*

Form 13: Kick with the Right Heel.

(1) Rotate the waist slightly to the right and cross the left hand over the right wrist.

(2) Move the left foot forward and shift your body weight to center to the left leg. Separate hands, rotating each hand in a large circle -- outward, down and back up until they join at the wrist. Both palms face inwards with the right hand in front of the left hand.

Points to follow: Keep your balance. Wrists are at shoulder level when hands are separated.

**Dragon Reaching**

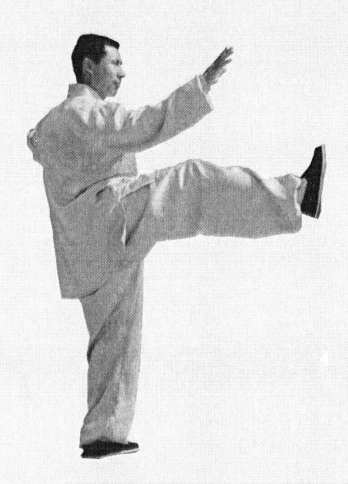

(3) Extend the arms sideways keeping them at shoulder level. Slowly lift the right foot and kick outward toward the southeast.

Points to follow: When kicking right foot, left leg is slightly bent. The kicking force should be focused on heel with the toe pointed up. The separation of hands should be coordinated with the kick. Right arm is parallel with right leg.

**Group Four**

*Form 14: Strike Ears with Both Fists*

Form 14: Double Wind Strike the Opponent's Ears with Both Fists.

(1) Following the right heel kick, draw the right leg back and while pulling both arms downward to the waist with the palms upward. Face south-east.

(2) Step out the right foot and shift the body weight on to the right leg resting in a right bow stance. At the same time, change both hands become fists, and strike as if aiming for an opponent's ears.

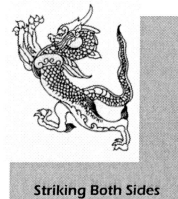

**Striking Both Sides**

Points to remember: Hold head and neck erect. Keep the waist and hips relaxed, and keep fists loosely clenched. Sink the shoulders and elbows. Arms are rounded.

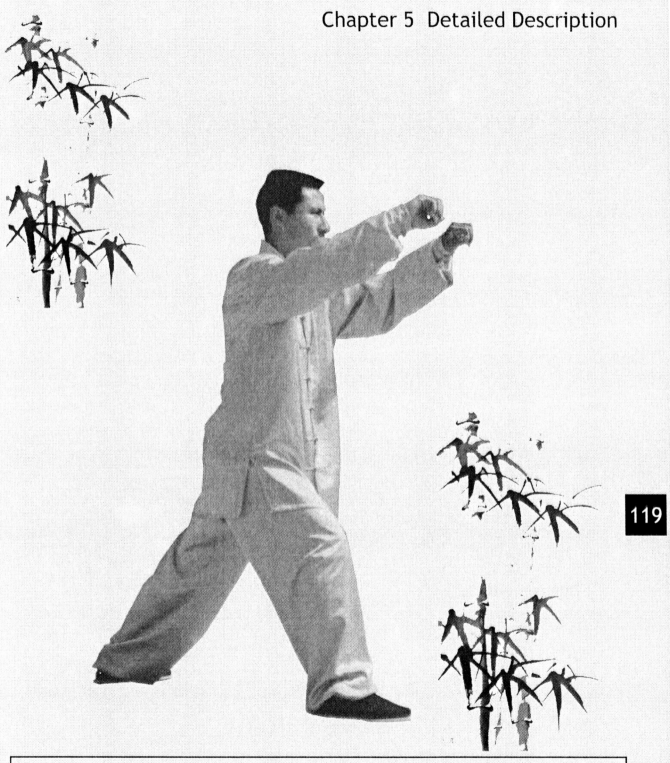

**Group Four**

## *Form 15: Turn and Kick with Left Heel*

Form 15: Turn and Kick with the Left Heel.

(1) Shift the body weight onto the left leg. Turn the right foot inward and turn the waist to the left. Shift the body center back to the right leg and sit on the right leg. Circle both arms downward and then up, crossing the wrists in front of the chest. Look towards the northwest.

**120**

(2) Lift the left foot and kick out with the left heel while extending both arms outward to shoulder level. Look toward the northwest.

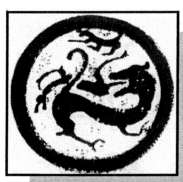

**Turning is Coming**

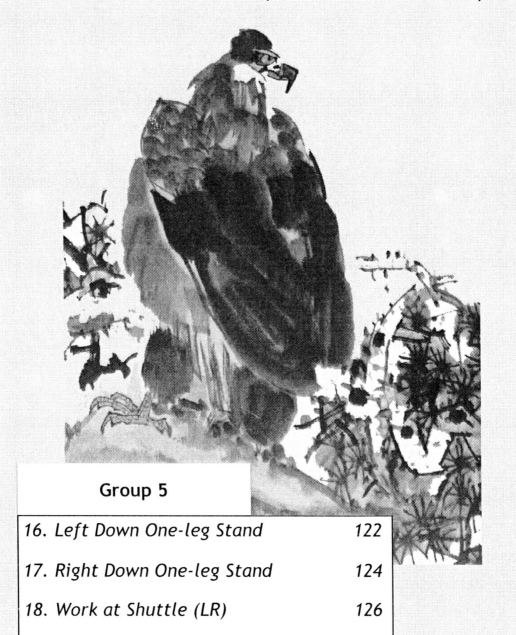

## Group 5

**Group Five**

*Form 16: Left Down One-leg Stand*

Form 16: Push Down then Stand on Left Leg (Left Golden Cock).

(1) After the left heel kick, draw back the left leg while changing the right hand into a hook. The left arm move back so the left hand comes to rest inside the right elbow. Look at the right hand.

(2) Bend down slowly on the right leg and stretch the left leg to the left keeping with the left toes inward. At the same time the left arm move downward keeping parallel to the side of left leg. Look at the left hand.

(3) Pivot on the left heel. Shift the body forward and up. Slowly move your weight to the left leg and form a left bow stance. Your left arm is now in front of your upper body, and your right arm with the hooked hand is behind your body.

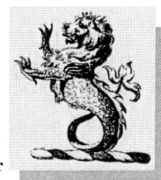

**Beast at Sea**

(4) Move your weight completely onto the left leg and draw the right leg up by bending the right knee. At the same time, press down the left hand down to the waist and lift the right hand up to ear level. Face west.

Points to follow: When bending down, turn toes of right foot outward and straighten left leg with the toes turned inward. The soles of both feet are flat on floor. Keep the torso upright. Bend the supporting leg slightly. Toes of the raised leg should point naturally downward. Relax the waist and sink the shoulders. Keep the torso erect.

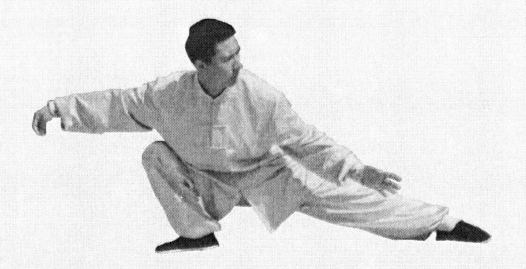

**Group Five**

*Form 17: Right Down One-leg*

*Stand*

Form 17: Push Down then Stand on Right Leg
(Right Golden Cock).

(1)  Put the right foot down with the toes touching the floor and pivot on the left heel. Rotate the body to the left. Raise the left hand up level with the ear and form a hook with the hand. The right hand moves toward the left arm coming to rest just inside the left elbow.

(2) Bend down slowly on the left leg and stretch the right leg to the right. The right toes point inward. Move the right arm down keeping it parallel to the inside of the right leg. Look at the right hand.

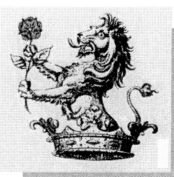

**Standing is Defending**

(3) Pivot on the right heel. Shift the body forward and up. Slowly move your weight to the right leg and form a right bow stance. Your right arm is now in front of your

upper body, and your left arm with the hooked hand is behind your body.

(4) Move your weight completely onto the right leg and draw the left leg up by bending the left knee. At the same time, press the right hand down to the waist and lift the left hand up to ear level. Face west.

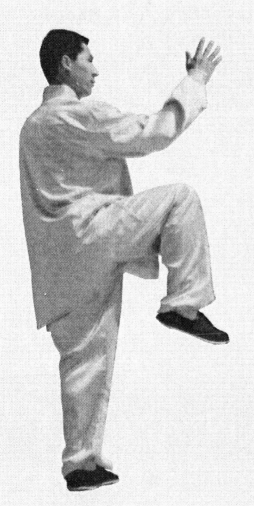

Points to follow: Raise the right foot slightly before bending down and moving the right leg sideways. Relax the waist and sink the shoulders. Keep the torso erect.

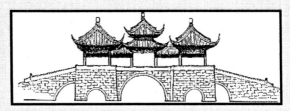

**Group Five**

*Form 18: Works at Shuttles*

Form 18: Fair Lady Works at Shuttles (Left and Right Sides).

(1) Step forward on your left foot; shift your body weight onto the left leg. Draw your right foot forward in such that the toes touch the ground beside your left foot. At the same time,

your arms hold a large ball in front of your chest with the left hand above the right. Face the south.

(2) Rotate your waist to the right and place your right foot forward with the right heel touching the ground first. Then shift 70% of your body weight onto the right leg and from a right bow stance. At the same time, rotate the right arm up so the hand is level with your forehead and

**Shifting is Balancing**

the palm faces out. Face the northwest.

(3) Shift your body weight back to the left leg, and rotate your waist slightly to the right. Shift your body weight back to the right leg, drawing your left foot up to rest beside your right foot with the toes touching the ground. At the same time, both arms hold a large ball in front of your chest with the right hand above the left. Face north.

(4) Rotate your waist to the left and place your left foot forward with the left heel touching the ground first. Then shift 70% of the body weight onto the front leg forming a left bow stance. At the same time, rotate the left arm up so the hand is level with your forehead and the palm faces out. Face southwest.

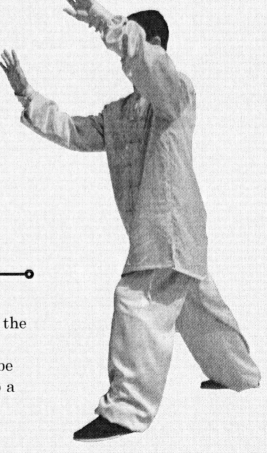

127

Points to follow: Do not lean forward when pushing hands forward. Do not the raise shoulders when moving hands upward. Movements of hands should be coordinated with waist and legs. Keep a transverse distance of about 30cm between heels while in a bow stance.

## Group Five

### *Form 19: Find a Needle at Sea Bottom*

In Form 19, we crouch down as if we were to find a needle at the bottom of the sea.

(1) Shift your body weight forward onto the left leg. Shift your body weight back to the right leg and bend the right knee. Raise the left foot slightly so the toes touch the ground. At the same time, the right arm circles down and then up, past the ear, and points down with the fingers.

**128**

Points to follow: Do not lean to far forward. Keep the buttocks tucked in. The left leg is slightly bent. Relax the waist.

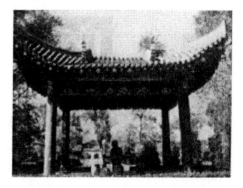

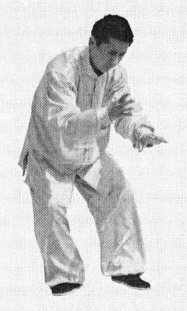

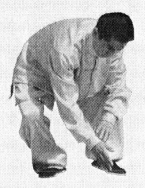

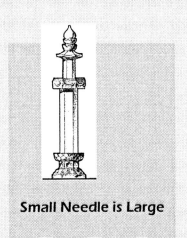

**Small Needle is Large**

**Group Five**

*Form 20: Flash Arms*

Form 20: Flash Arms or Fan through the Arms.

(1) Move the right arm up just above your forehead. At the same time, lift the left palm up to guard the right wrist. Your hands now form a cross level with

your forehead. Shift your body weight forward into a left bow stance. Push the left palm forward and turn the right palm outward and slightly up. Face west.

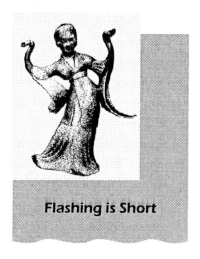

**Flashing is Short**

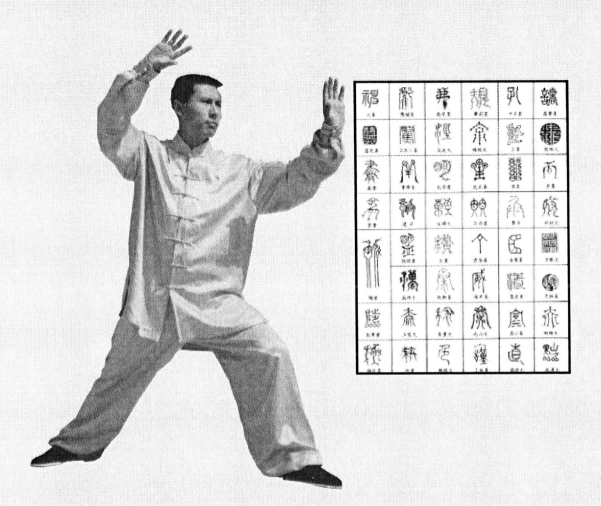

Points to follow: Do not straighten arm when you push left palm forward. Coordinate the pushing of the hands with the movement left bow stance. Relax the waist and sink the shoulders. Keep the torso upright.

132

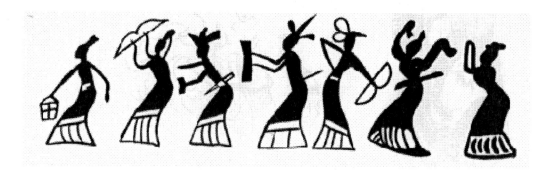

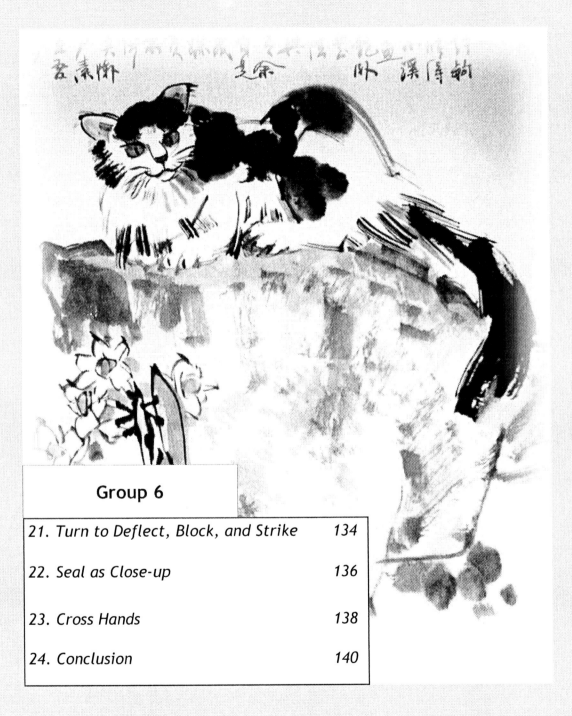

## Group 6

**Group Six**

## *Form 21: Turn to Deflect, Block and Strike*

Three distinctive moves are performed in Form 21: (1) turn to deflect, (2) block as if someone were throwing a punch at you, and (3) punch. This is time we strike back.

(1) Shift your body weight to the right leg. Pivot on the left heel with the toes turning inward. Then shift your center back onto the left leg while lowering both arms in a large circle with

the left arm above the right arm. Your right hand forms a fist. Draw the right foot back next to the left foot. Face north.

(2) Rotate the body to the right while stepping the right foot forward. Then shift the center completely onto the right leg drawing the left foot to the side of the right foot. At the same time, the right

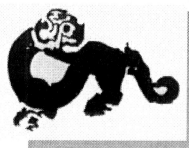

**Turning is to Deflect**

fist rotates in front of the body and the left arm rotates in a large circle in front of the

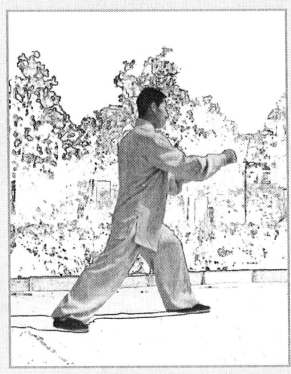

front body. Face south.

(3)      Step your left foot forward forming a left bow stance. Pull back the left hand so the palm guards the inside of the right elbow. Punch the right fist forward.  Face east.

135

Points to follow: Hold the right fist loosely. Draw front arm inward and rest it by the right side of the waist, palm upward. The right shoulder follows the punch, extending forward slightly. Sink the shoulders and elbows and keep the right arm slightly bent. Relax the waist and keep the body upright.

## Group Six

### *Form 22: Seal as Close-up*

The name of Form 22 is to convey a message that one seals off the pathway of incoming strike as if closing a door.

(1) Turn your body slightly to the right and sit back on the right leg. At the same time, lower the left hand to beneath the right elbow and

**136**

open the right fist. Both palm face up. Separate both arms until they are about shoulder width apart, pull both hands back to the chest and down to chest level. Push both hands forward while shifting your body weight forward into a left bow stance. Face east.

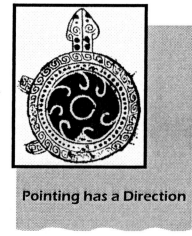

**Pointing has a Direction**

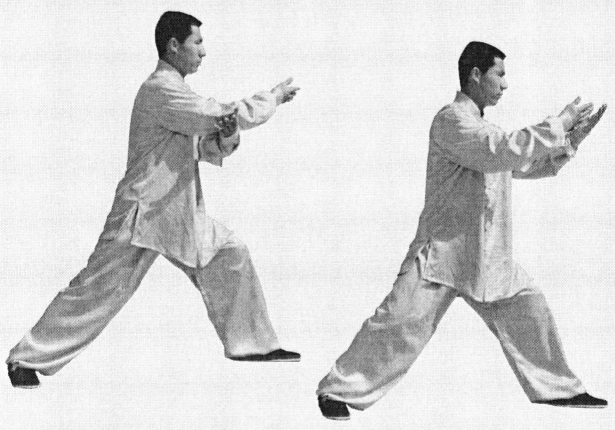

Points to follow: When sitting back, do not lean backward or let the buttocks protrude. Do not pull arms straight back, keep them curved. Relax your shoulders and turn elbows slightly outward. Hands should be no farther than shoulder width apart when pushing forward. Keep your body upright.

## Group Six

### *Form 23: Cross Hands*

Form 23: Cross Hands.

(1) Sit back on the right leg and rotate the body to the right while turning the left foot inward so both toes facing the south. At the same time, circle the right arm down.

(2) Shift the body weight back onto the left leg while circling both arms down and then up so both palms are crossed at the wrist in front of the chest. Palms face inward. At the same time, draw the right foot in so it is parallel with the left foot and feet are shoulder width apart. Bend your knees slightly. Face south.

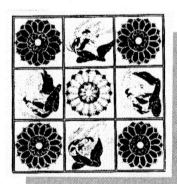

**Turning Makes a Circle**

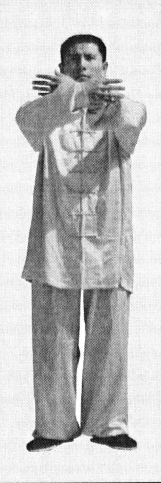

Points to follow: Do not lean forward when separating or crossing hands. Keep arms rounded in a comfortable position. Keep torso erect and sink shoulders and elbows down. Fingers are slightly curved. Body weight is equally distributed between legs. While bending knees, keep the waist relaxed and buttocks slightly pulled in.

**Group Six**

*Form 24: Conclusion*

Form 24 is the finishing form.

(1) Separate your hands and raise both arms forward. Lower the hand and rest them beside your hips. Move the left next to the right leg. Face south.

Points to remember: Allow your arms to hang at your sides. Keep your neck and back straight and upright. Keep you chin slightly tucked in. Your eyes are concentrated and full of spirit. Sink the chest and keep the back rounded. Your body is centered and upright. Keep the whole body relaxed.

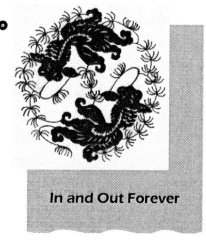

**In and Out Forever**

# Chapter 5  Detailed Description

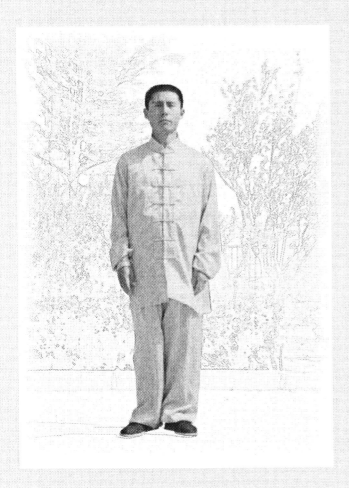

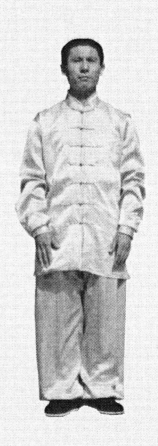

141

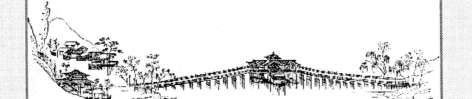

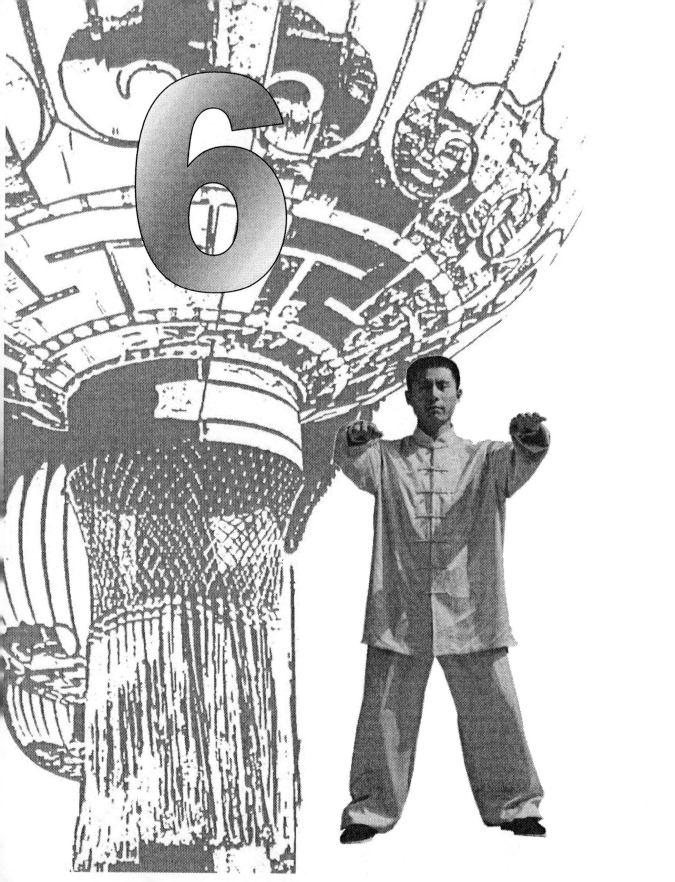

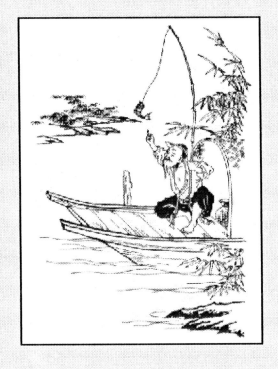

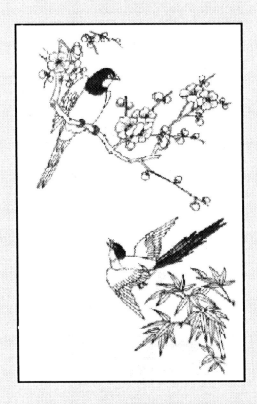

In this chapter, several groups of questions will be answered. They are the questions collected from Tai Chi classes, some of which were from beginners and some were asked by students who have practiced a year or more and gained deeper understanding of the principles of Tai Chi. These questions and answers will help you see how others understand Tai Chi as an art of health exercise.

# Tai Chi for Health

*Questions*

1. What kind of clothes and shoes should Tai Chi practitioners wear?

2. How much time should be spent practicing Tai Chi each day?

3. How to judge the quality of a person's Tai Chi Chuan?

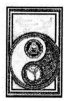

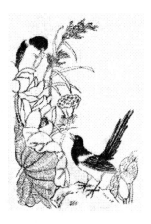

144

## Answers

Q:  What kind of clothes and shoes should tai chi practitioners wear?

A:  Loosely fitting clothes and soft flat shoes, such as sneakers, will do.

Q:  How much time should be spent practicing tai chi each day?

A:  It depends. One must feel comfortable at the end of practice and not tired. One must not exercise too much.

Q:  How to judge the quality of a person's Tai Chi Chuan?

A:  To tell the quality of a person's tai chi form, just examine the following:

(1) The angles of the body when performing each posture and the transitions between each movement; (2) the pace of the movements; (3) the height of each posture. A person is considered a good practitioner when he/she can carry out every movement gracefully, with coordination and precision. A good tai chi practitioner keeps the same height during the execution of the forms. He/she does not bob up and down. The ending form finishes in the place the opening form began. The form is practiced in a constant and regular pace. The movements of the limbs should be coordinated with the waist. All postures should be erect, coordinated, continuous, flowing, and balanced throughout the forms. The whole body should be relaxed.

# Tai Chi for Health

> **Question**
>
> What are the general principles in practicing Tai Chi Chuan?

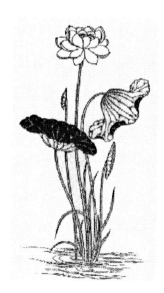

*The following rules are attributed to master Yang Chengfu: Tai Chi Chuan 10 Important Points.*

1. The spirit at the top of the head should be light and sensitive.
2. Sink the chest and raise the back.
3. Relax the waist.
4. Distinguish full and empty (substantial and insubstantial).
5. Sink the shoulders and drop the elbows.
6. Use mind not strength.
7. Coordination between the upper and lower body.
8. Internal and external unity.
9. Continuity without stopping.
10. Seeking stillness in movement.

## *Answer*

Q:   What are the general principles in practicing Tai Chi Chuan?

A:   In general, tai chi practitioner should follow the following rules:

1. The head energy insubstantially leads upward.

2. The eyes gaze with concentration.

3. Keep the chest in and raise back.

4. Sink the shoulders and drop the elbows lightly.

5. Keep body center straight, central, and upright.

6. Relax waist and thighs.

7. Both feet flat on the floor.

8. The top and bottom of the body are coordinated in a harmonized way.

9. Distinguish between fullness and emptiness.

10. Internal and external are harmonized with natural breathing.

11. Mind leads, not straight force.

12. All postures flow smoothly, the entire body is comfortable.

13. All postures should be centered and upright.

14. Keep stillness in motion and motion in stillness.

# Tai Chi for Health

*Questions*

1. Some people say: "The head energy in-substantially leads upward," what does it mean?

2. How do I understand the meaning that "The eyes gaze with concentration"?

3. Do I need to "Keep the chest in and raise the back lightly"?

4. Why do I have to "Lower and sink the shoulders and drop the elbows"?

5. Why do I need to "Keep body center straight, central, and upright"?

6. What am I exactly doing when they tell me to "Relax waist and thighs"?

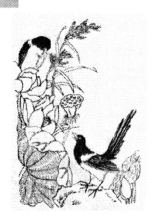

148

## Answers

Q:   When people say: "The head energy insubstantially leads upward," what does mean?

A:   The head feels like it is suspended from above. In this way, the whole body moves lightly and agilely.

Q:   How do I understand the meaning that "the eyes gaze with concentration"?

A:   When a person's mind has concentrated, he/she will be able to aware even the slightest movement.

Q:   Do I need to "Keep the chest in and raise the back lightly"?

A:   The back has the feeling of being lifted lightly, and the chest is the slightly sunken. In this way, your chest is relaxed and the lungs move freely.

Q:   Why do I have to "Lower and sink the shoulders and drop the elbows"?

A:   Lowering the shoulders and dropping elbows helps with relaxation. This makes the transition easy.

Q:   Why do I need to "Keep body center straight, central, and upright"?

A:   The body's spine should be straight and erect, not leaning to the side.

**149**

Q:   What am I exactly doing when they tell me to "Relax waist and thighs"?

A:   The waist commands all movements. Relaxation of your waist and thighs will make the connection between the waist and the knees easy.

# Tai Chi for Health

*Questions*

1. Why do I have to put "both feet flat on the floor"?

2. What is the meaning that "the top and bottom of the body are coordinated in a harmonized way"?

3. Why do I have to "distinguish fullness and emptiness"?

4. How do I understand that "mind leads, not straight force"?

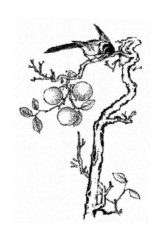

## Answers

Q:  Why do I have to put "both feet flat on the floor"?

A:  The feet (or foot) must always be flat, sticky on the ground and relaxed, This is so that your body center will be rooted.

Q:  What is the meaning that "the top and bottom of the body are coordinated in a harmonized way"?

A:  The entire body must move in an integrated, coordinated way. Follow three harmonies: hands with feet; shoulders with limbs; elbows with knees.

Q:  Why do I have to "distinguish fullness and emptiness"?

A:  If one leg bears the major body weight, it is full, otherwise, it is empty.

Q:  How do I understand that "mind leads, not straight force"?

A:  This means you should think first before you move into the postures.

**151**

# Tai Chi for Health

*Questions*

1. Why do some people tell me that "all postures flow smoothly, the entire body is comfortable"?

2. What is the meaning that "all postures should be centered and upright"?

3. It seems contradictory to "keep stillness in motion and motion in stillness", doesn't it?

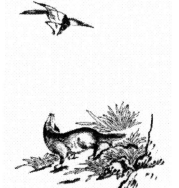

## Answers

Q:  Why do some people tell me that "all postures flow smoothly, the entire body is comfortable"?

A:  The whole forms should be performed smoothly from the beginning to the end. There should be no breaks, jerks, or sharp angles. All movements should be natural and comfortable.

Q:  What is the meaning that "all postures should be centered and upright"?

A:  Your body should be upright, centered, balanced and coordinated. Your arms and legs should be neither too extended nor shrunken in.

Q:  It seems contradictory to "keep stillness in motion and motion in stillness", doesn't it?

A:  This means all movements are peaceful and flowing.

153

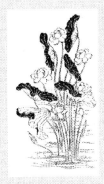

*Question*

How to breathe while practicing tai chi forms?

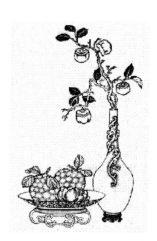

154

## Answer

Q:   How to breathe while practicing tai chi forms?

A:   Breath naturally.  After training for a long time, one should be able to breathe according to the following rules with each posture:

1. open (inhale) and close (exhale);

2. up (inhale) and down (exhale);

3. raise (inhale) and sink (exhale);

4. back (inhale) and out (exhale);

5. squeeze (inhale) and extend (exhale);

6. shrink (inhale) and stretch (exhale).

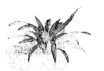

155

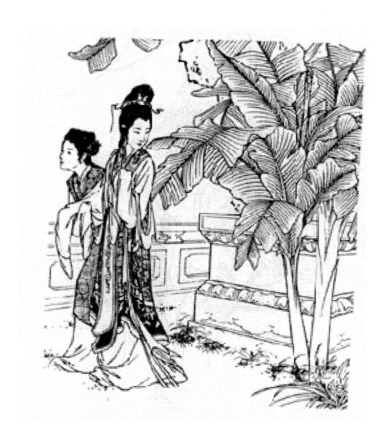

# Reference:

1. Tai Chi Chuan Sports, edited by People's Republic of China Physical Education Committee, Beijing China 1996. ISBN:7-5009-1150-5

2. How to Best Learn the 24 Simplified Tai Chi Chuan, Zhang Qi Hua and Lu Ping, People's Physical Education Publishing House, China 2000. ISBN 7-5009-1703-1

3. The Encyclopedia of Tai Chi Chuan, Feng Zhigang and Li Binci, Education Yard Publishing House, Beijing, China 2005. ISBN 7-5077-1170-6.

4. Tai Chi: Yang Family Basic 24 Forms (Book and DVD), Li Huilin, Da Lian Audio and Visual Publishing House, China 2005. ISRC CN-D03-05-0061-0/V-J7.

5. The 24 Simplified Forms of Tai Chi Chuan, Li Deyin, The Audio and Visual Publishing House of Beijing TV Art Center, Beijing, China 2005. ISRC CN-C07-02-318-00/V.G4.

# Monthly Workout

| Sun | Mon | Tue | Wed | Thu | Fri | Sat |
|-----|-----|-----|-----|-----|-----|-----|
|     |     |     |     |     |     |     |
|     |     |     |     |     |     |     |
|     |     |     |     |     |     |     |
|     |     |     |     |     |     |     |
|     |     |     |     |     |     |     |

Tai Chi for Health

# MONTHLY WORKOUT

| Sun | Mon | Tue | Wed | Thu | Fri | Sat |
|-----|-----|-----|-----|-----|-----|-----|
|     |     |     |     |     |     |     |
|     |     |     |     |     |     |     |
|     |     |     |     |     |     |     |
|     |     |     |     |     |     |     |

## Plan your workout

It is a good idea to plan out your monthly workout schedule with your teacher at some point of your class so that you do not miss any class. Use the calendar templates here to mark your schedule or photo copy them for your class.

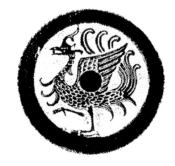

# Tai Chi Accessory Order Form

| Item # | Description | Qty. | Price | Subtotal |
|--------|-------------|------|-------|----------|
|        |             |      |       |          |
|        |             |      |       |          |
|        |             |      |       |          |
|        |             |      |       |          |
|        |             |      |       |          |
|        |             |      |       |          |

Order total: _____

Tax: _____

Shipping: _____

Total: _____

Name _____

Address _____

_____

_____

_____

Phone _____

Method of Payment

☐ Check

☐ Bill Me

☐ Visa

☐ MasterCard

☐ American Express

Credit Card # _____ Exp. date _____

Signature _____

# Appendix B: Order Forms and Coupon Templates

| Name | | | | |
|---|---|---|---|---|
| Address | Sign up for: | | Time | Price |

Method of Payment

☐ Bill Me     ☐ Visa

☐ Check     ☐ MasterCard

☐ American Express

Phone

Credit Card #     Exp. date

Signature

Subtotal: _____

Tax: _____

Total: _____

---

## First Time Student
## 10% OFF

Valid after Purchasing the TAI CHI for Health book

Phone:

Expiration Date:

---

## Tai Chi Class Consultation

**Valid for Participating Clubs**

Phone:

Expiration Date:

---

## Special Offer

Teachers may use this book for Tai Chi classes. Tai Chi clothes or other teaching materials may be ordered from the TAI CHI instructors using the forms provided here. As a way of assisting Tai Chi teachers, two coupons are printed here for the promotional purpose of any Tai Chi classes.

Write to Dr. Cheng Zhao about Tai Chi if you have any questions and comments.

Write to Dr. Cheng Zhao about Tai Chi if you have any questions and comments.

309 Woodbine Drive
Terre Haute, IN 47803
U.S.A.
Phone: 812-877-6328
E-mail: taichi.cheng@gmail.com

**Agilceed books**
*Knowledge changes life*

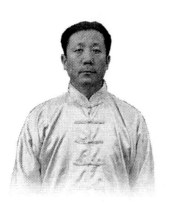

Agilceed books is a small publishing company promoting the share and exchange of the knowledge that positively affects people's life. Agilceed books firmly believes that the personal ownership of knowledge will be more meaningful after the knowledge has been expressed clearly and systematically in public and reaches the people who need it. Agilceed book will continue to help people to publish their knowledge in the right way.

## About Dr. Cheng Zhao

Dr. Cheng Zhao is a full professor at Indiana State University. He started his formal Tai Chi Chuan training more than 20 years ago in China. In 1987, he became a disciple of grandmaster Xin Yu He. Coincidentally, Li Guang Qi and Dr. Zhao were in the same class on the same day. Cheng Zhao continues to learn and practice Yang style (Xin group) Tai Chi since then. To meet the interests of Tai Chi practitioners in Terre Haute area in Indiana, Dr. Zhao founded Indiana Tai Chi Academy in 2005. He currently leads a group of Tai Chi practitioners to learn and practice Tai Chi Standard Forms; Tai Chi 24 Hand Forms; Tai Chi 32 Sword Forms; Basic Tai Chi Pushing Hand Forms; Traditional Yang Style (Xin Group) Long/Short Forms. He hopes through his teaching, many people could experience the art of Tai Chi and discover a genuine path for health and tranquility.

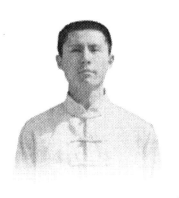

Li Guang Qi became a disciple of Grandmaster Xin Yu He in 1987. He followed Xin Yu He for 11 years and has taught and practiced Tai Chi in Jinan, Shandong of China for more than 20 years. He inherited and developed all grandmaster Xin style Tai Chi training. In this book, we would like to thank Master Li Guang Qi for allowing us to publish his Tai Chi pictures and his performance DVD for the first time.

Yang Style Tai Chi

Yang style Tai Chi was founded by Yang Lu Chan (1799-1872). His grandson, Yang Cheng Fu (1883-1936) is the third generation of the Yang family. He taught many Tai Chi students who later became famous. One of Yang Cheng Fu's leading disciple was Li Ya Xuan (1894 - 1976). Li's famous disciple was Liu Zhong Qiao whose last disciple was Xin Yu He. Master Xin spent 9 years learning Tai Chi from Liu Zhong Qiao and reached a very high level in Yang style Tai Chi at the end of class. He founded his Yang style (Xin group) Tai Chi in Jinan, Shandong Province of China. The current leader of Xin group Tai Chi is Master Li Guang Qi.

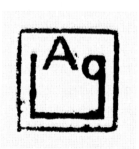

| | |
|---|---|
| ISBN | 0-976118-31-9 |
| SIZE | 7.5" x 9.25" |
| EDITION | 1st. Ed. V3-63250 |
| MANF | TAIC-319 |
| PUB DATE | 2006-3-17 |
| TRACK NO. | V5-65110 |

Printed in the United States
52790LVS00004B/35